D0270898

OXFORD BROOKES UNIVERSITY LIBRARY
Harcourt Hill
A fine will be levied if this item becomes
overdue. ~~To renew please ring 01865 483133~~
(reserved items cannot be renewed).
Harcourt Hill enquiries 01865 488222
www.brookes.ac.uk/services/library

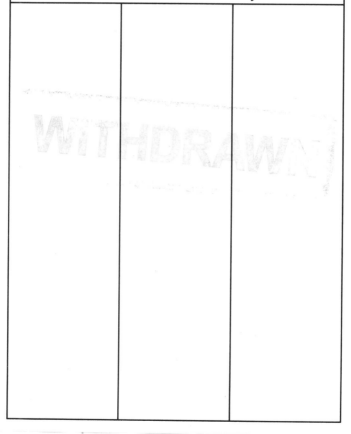

LIBRARY

00 964276 06

The Material Child

Growing Up in Consumer Culture

DAVID BUCKINGHAM

polity

Copyright © David Buckingham 2011

The right of David Buckingham to be identified as Author of this Work has been asserted in accordance with the UK Copyright, Designs and Patents Act 1988.

First published in 2011 by Polity Press

Reprinted 2012

Polity Press
65 Bridge Street
Cambridge CB2 1UR, UK

Polity Press
350 Main Street
Malden, MA 02148, USA

All rights reserved. Except for the quotation of short passages for the purpose of criticism and review, no part of this publication may be reproduced, stored in a retrieval system, or transmitted, in any form or by any means, electronic, mechanical, photocopying, recording or otherwise, without the prior permission of the publisher.

ISBN-13: 978-0-7456-4770-8
ISBN-13: 978-0-7456-4771-5(pb)

A catalogue record for this book is available from the British Library.

Typeset in 11.25 on 13 pt Dante
by Toppan Best-set Premedia Limited
Printed and bound in Great Britain by MPG Books Group Limited, Bodmin, Cornwall

The publisher has used its best endeavours to ensure that the URLs for external websites referred to in this book are correct and active at the time of going to press. However, the publisher has no responsibility for the websites and can make no guarantee that a site will remain live or that the content is or will remain appropriate.

Every effort has been made to trace all copyright holders, but if any have been inadvertently overlooked the publisher will be pleased to include any necessary credits in any subsequent reprint or edition.

For further information on Polity, visit our website: www.politybooks.com

ACC. NO. 964276 06		FUND HDEC
LOC. ET	CATEGORY STAN	PRICE £15.99
07 JUN 2013		
CLASS No. 306.3083 BUC		
OXFORD BROOKES UNIVERSITY LIBRARY		

Contents

Acknowledgements

In April 2008, I was invited by two UK government departments (the Department of Children, Schools and Families (DCSF), and the Department of Culture, Media and Sport (DCMS) to lead an independent assessment of 'the impact of the commercial world on children's wellbeing'. The assessment report was finally (and belatedly) published in December 2009, in the dying days of Gordon Brown's Labour government; and at the time of writing, it can still be accessed (along with a range of supplementary reports and materials) on the Department for Education website. This book has partly emerged from the work of the assessment, and it incorporates some material first written for the report. I would like to thank the extremely distinguished group of academic colleagues who worked on the assessment with me: Paddy Barwise, Hugh Cunningham, Mary Jane Kehily, Sonia Livingstone, Mary MacLeod, Lydia Martens, Ginny Morrow, Agnes Nairn and Brian Young. I am absolutely certain that they would not endorse every word I have written here; but I am nevertheless very grateful to them for their expert and often challenging input. I am also grateful to the colleagues from the University of Loughborough, the Open University, Stirling University and the Social Issues Research Centre who produced the literature reviews on which I have continued to rely here. Perhaps my greatest debt, however, is to Jane Geraghty of the DCSF, who managed to keep me reasonably sane throughout the process, and helped me to learn a good deal about the workings of government along the way. Responsibility for the arguments presented here remains my own.

I would also like to thank my colleagues in various institutions with whom I have worked on these issues over the past several years: Rebekah Willett and Shakuntala Banaji at the Institute of Education; Vebjørg Tingstad, Tora Korsvold and Ingunn Hagen at the Norwegian Centre for Child Research; and Sara Bragg at the Open University. I am also grateful to various institutions and organizations for offering me opportunities to speak on these topics over the past couple of years, and for their feedback, especially: OMEP in Athens (Litsa Kourti); the Open University (Mary Jane Kehily, Rachel Thomson and Liz McFall); Syracuse University (Sari Biklen); Sheffield University (Allison James); Goldsmiths College (Angela McRobbie); the School of Oriental and African Studies (Annabelle Sreberny and Mark Hobart); the 'Onscenity' research network (Feona Attwood); the Copenhagen Business School (Birgitte Tufte); the University of Ghent (Daniel Biltereyst); and the 'Colloque Enfance et Cultures' in Paris (Regine Sirota and Sylvie Octobre). I would also like to thank Vebjørg Tingstad, Martyn Richmond and two anonymous reviewers for their comments on the manuscript; and the staff at Polity, especially Andrea Drugan and Lauren Mulholland, for their support.

Introduction

Over the past decade, the figure of the child consumer has been the focus of increasing attention and debate. On the one hand, children have become more and more important (and indeed lucrative) both as a market in their own right and as a means to reach adult markets. Companies are using a much wider range of marketing techniques, which go well beyond conventional advertising; and they are targeting children directly at an ever-younger age. Marketers often claim that children are becoming 'empowered' in this new commercial environment: the market is seen to be responding to needs and desires on the part of children that have hitherto been largely ignored or marginalized, not least because of the social dominance of adults.

Yet, on the other hand, there is a growing number of popular publications bemoaning the apparent 'commercialization' of childhood. This argument seems to presume that children used to live in an essentially non-commercial world; and that their entry into the marketplace over the past several decades has had a wide range of negative consequences for their wellbeing. Commercialization is seen to cause harm to many aspects of children's physical and mental health, as well as generating concerns about issues such as 'sexualization' and 'materialism'. Such campaigning publications typically regard children not as empowered, but rather as powerless victims of commercial manipulation and exploitation.

Furthermore, as we shall see, many critics claim that a 'consumerist' orientation now pervades all aspects of the social world in capitalist societies, and that users of non-commercial services such as health and education are increasingly positioned (and have come to see themselves) as consumers. Yet children are also likely to be surrounded by messages about the dangers of consumerism and materialism and by exhortations to recycle or to enjoy what is 'free' in life, such as friendship or nature – often paradoxically purveyed by commercial media themselves.

This book seeks to refute the popular view of children as incompetent and vulnerable consumers that is espoused by many of the campaigners;

but it also rejects the celebratory account of consumption as an expression of children's power and autonomy. Rather, it aims to challenge the terms in which the social issue of children's consumption is typically framed and understood; and in the process, to question how human agency and identity are experienced in late modern 'consumer societies'. To see children's role in the consumer market simply in terms of a dyadic relationship between children and marketers – whether we see that relationship as one of manipulation or of empowerment – is to oversimplify the issue.

Instead, I propose a view of children's consumption as inextricably embedded within wider networks of social relationships; and I argue that, in modern industrial (and 'post industrial') societies, consumption is a domain both of constraint and control, and of choice and creativity. This approach, I suggest, takes us beyond the moralistic and sentimental views about children's consumption that tend to dominate the public debate. It also helps us to recognize some of the ironies and complexities of contemporary consumer culture, and particularly of the more 'interactive' or 'participatory' forms that are currently emerging.

I understand 'consumption' in broad terms. Consumption is not just about the purchasing of goods, but also about the ways in which they are used, appropriated and adapted, both individually and collectively. It is not just about goods, but also about services – not just about what you possess, but also about what you are able to do. Studying children's consumption means looking not only at advertising and marketing, but also at the many other ways in which commercial forces and market relations affect children's environment and their social and cultural experiences. It is not only about toys or clothes or food, but also about media, about leisure and about education. Ultimately, it is not just about objects or commodities, but also about social meanings and pleasures.

It is for these reasons that I talk about consumer *culture*, and not just about consumption. The term 'culture' is, of course, a complex and loaded one; but for me it implies a fundamental interest in how meanings are created within a given social context, and in consumption as a means of communicating or signifying meaning. As Don Slater (1997: 8) puts it, 'consumer culture denotes a social arrangement in which the relation between lived culture and social resources, between meaningful ways of life and the symbolic and material resources on which they depend, is mediated through markets'. From this perspective, we would need to resist the simple opposition between commerce and culture on which a great deal of discussion of this issue is premised. This is particularly true of children: as Dan Cook (2004) has argued, the relation between children and the market is frequently seen in terms of the relation between the sacred and the profane – an opposition which makes the discussion of 'children's consumer culture' appear almost sacrilegious.

This emphasis on meaning and communication is not, of course, to imply that consumers are autonomous or all-powerful, or that they can make any meanings they choose: commercial producers and marketers obviously set constraints and parameters, and provide and shape the resources that make consumption possible. Social relationships construct and mediate consumer culture, yet consumer culture in turn shapes the nature and meaning of social relationships. As we shall see, this is a complex dynamic, whose consequences are often unpredictable and hard to pin down.

Even so, this is not a book about the *commercialization* of childhood. Commercial influences do not impinge upon or invade childhood as if from outside; nor are they an inexorable force that entirely determines children's experiences. Rather, contemporary childhood takes place in and through market relations – as indeed it has done for centuries. Ultimately, consumption is part of the lived experience of capitalism; and children do not stand outside that, in some pure or unsullied space, even if that is what some commentators appear to imagine or wish.

The first three chapters provide the theoretical grounding for the book as a whole. Chapter 1 reviews the popular debate about children's consumption, contrasting the rhetoric of the campaigners with that of the new wave of children's marketers. Chapter 2 introduces theories of consumption as they have been developed largely in relation to adults, while chapter 3 looks at the various ways in which children's consumption has been addressed in theory and research. Collectively, these chapters argue for a broader socio-cultural approach to children's consumption that moves beyond the simple polarization introduced above.

Chapters 4 and 5 look, respectively, at the history of children's consumption, and at the contemporary children's market. These chapters point to some considerable continuities here, both in the strategies adopted by marketers and in the ambivalence with which they are viewed by parents and children. However, they also point to some significant shifts in the children's market, not least with the emergence of digital marketing, and discuss some of the ethical problems they raise.

Chapters 6 and 7 provide a critical analysis of two key concerns in the recent debate about children's consumption, namely obesity and 'sexualization'. These chapters challenge the terms in which these issues have been framed both within the public debate and within psychological research, and counterpose some of the rhetoric with evidence from empirical studies with children themselves.

Chapters 8 and 9 explore two aspects of the social relationships in which children's consumption occurs: namely, relationships with parents and with peers. Here again, I seek to challenge some of the terms in which these issues are understood – for example in popular labels like 'pester power' and 'peer pressure'. I also seek to provide an alternative to views of children's consumption that see it as a simple matter of cause-and-effect.

In chapters 10 and 11, the attention shifts away from consumption itself to focus on the ways in which market relations shape children's experiences more broadly. These chapters focus on two areas – children's television and education – that in recent years have increasingly come to be led by commercial interests and commercial models. As I suggest, these developments have had some significant, albeit ambivalent, consequences for children in particular.

Chapter 12 is a brief conclusion, which picks up a theme that serves as a running thread throughout the book, and particularly through the latter chapters: this is the issue of inequality. I argue that a consumer society tends to exacerbate some of the negative consequences of inequality; but that simply regulating the activities of marketers is unlikely to make a significant difference to the broader structures that create inequality in the first place.

This book is intended to provide an overview of a complex and diverse field; but it is also a book with a definite standpoint. It draws on a wide range of research, some of which is necessarily dealt with in a very summary form. I hope that it will stimulate further work in this area, and contribute to a more informed and productive public debate about one of the most pressing and controversial issues of our times.

1

Exploited or empowered?
Constructing the child consumer

From the moment they are born, children today are already consumers. Contemporary childhoods are lived out in a world of commercial goods and services. Marketing to children is by no means new, but children now play an increasingly important role, both as consumers in their own right and as influences on parents. They are exposed to a growing number and range of commercial messages, which extend far beyond traditional media advertising. They are surrounded by invitations and inducements to buy and to consume; and commercial forces also increasingly impact on their experiences in areas such as public broadcasting, education and play.

Consumer culture offers children a wide range of opportunities and experiences that they would not have enjoyed in earlier times. Yet, far from being welcomed or celebrated, children's consumption has often been perceived as an urgent social problem. Politicians, religious leaders, child welfare campaigners and consumer rights groups – not to mention armies of newspaper columnists and media pundits – routinely express concern and outrage at the harmful influence of advertising and marketing on children. Such concern is not confined to a single moral or political perspective: traditional conservatives and anti-capitalist activists, feminists and religious fundamentalists, all join forces in a chorus of condemnation. Children, they argue, should be kept away from harmful commercial influences: advertising and marketing to children should be banned, and parents should seek to raise their children in a 'commercial-free' environment. In these debates, consumerism is often tied up with a series of other social problems. Advertising and marketing are blamed for causing obesity and eating disorders, for encouraging premature sexualization, for promoting materialistic values, and for inciting conflict within the family and the peer group. Consumerism, it would seem, is destroying the fundamental values of childhood – and, in the process, it is making children's and parents' lives a misery.

And yet the focus of the objections here is often far from clearly defined. 'Junk food' advertising, sexy underage fashion models and deceptive marketing online are all precise enough as targets. But the criticisms of consumerism and the commercial world often range much more broadly: indeed, the debate often seems to be about the wholesale destruction of childhood itself. So are we only talking about advertising and marketing here, or about the economic system as a whole? Is 'consumption' just about buying stuff, or about using it too? Where does 'the commercial world' begin and end – and where might we find a 'non-commercial world'? Does the act of consumption inevitably involve sets of values or ideologies, such as 'consumerism' or 'materialism' – and how are these to be identified? Why are certain kinds of consumption implicitly seen to be acceptable – buying books or classical music CDs, or paying for your children to attend ballet classes – while others are not? Is the problem one of *excessive* consumption, or of people having *too much* money to spend – and, if so, who defines what counts as 'too much'?

Such arguments are certainly applied to adults, yet they seem to carry a unique force when it comes to children. Parents are frequently urged to resist consumerism *on behalf of* their children: only then, it would seem, will children be able to experience a good or proper childhood. Yet on what basis are some consumer products perceived to be inappropriate for children in general, or for children at particular ages? Why are some things deemed acceptable for adults, and not for children? Are children in general somehow more vulnerable than adults to the harmful behaviours and values apparently promoted by consumer culture? In what sense is it even possible, in a modern capitalist society, for children to be kept away from commercial influences – and what might be the negative consequences of seeking to do so? What are the alternative values that somehow stand outside the commercial world, and which might enable children and parents to resist its influence?

The construction of social problems

These questions point to the fact that the 'problem' of the child consumer is typically defined in quite particular ways. At stake are assumptions both about consumption – about what consumption is, and about 'good' and 'bad' consumption – and about children – about what children essentially are or should be, and about 'good' and 'bad' childhoods. These assumptions are not given statements of fact, and they are not neutral. On the contrary, the figure of the child consumer is framed and constructed in specific ways, which thereby marginalize or prevent other ways of thinking about the issue.

In recent years, analyses of social problems have explored such questions from a 'social constructionist' perspective. Broadly speaking, social problems can be defined as phenomena that are believed to be morally wrong, and that are seen to require positive intervention. Yet the things we identify and categorize as social problems are not stable or fixed. On the contrary, problems are defined in different ways in different social and cultural settings, and people often disagree about how they should be understood. Problems or issues are not simply given, but actively constructed. Groups of people have to identify, select and name them: problems must be categorized and typified in particular ways in order to become the focus of public attention. The metaphor of 'framing' is often used here: putting a problem into a frame serves to define it and focus attention on it, but it also detracts attention away from what lies outside the frame, and thereby limits the ways in which we can understand the problem in the first place.

Social constructionists suggest that in the more diverse and fluid context of contemporary societies, there is less consensus about right and wrong; and, accordingly, the construction of social problems is often a contested process, in which feelings may increasingly come to count for more than logic or evidence (Loseke, 2003). The actions of 'claims-makers' play a central role in this process. Studies have explored how key claims-makers – campaigners, politicians, experts, media commentators – work to define a social problem and increase its public visibility, often in pursuit of their own sectional interests. This typically entails mobilizing forms of rhetoric. Claims-makers compete with each other for media attention, often by overstating the scale of the problem, focusing on dramatic or spectacular manifestations, and occasionally drawing on dubious expert or scientific evidence (Hilgartner and Bosk, 1988). Such claims are often cumulative and mutually reinforcing, and so the scope of the problem tends to expand. The claims with most power to persuade are those that reflect other dominant themes – and indeed stereotypes and prejudices – within the culture. Simple claims are more effective than complicated ones; and formulaic stories featuring 'goodies' and 'baddies' – often involving melodramatic narratives of corruption and decline – are less likely to be challenged, not least because they can invoke powerful emotions. This is most evidently the case with the generation of 'moral panics' – a phenomenon that has, of course, been the focus of a great deal of sociological and historical analysis (e.g. Barker, 1984; Cohen, 2002; Springhall, 1998).

The figure of the child – or perhaps a certain idea of childhood – is often crucial here. As Joel Best (1990, 1994) and others have noted, the contemporary rise to prominence of child abuse as a social issue can be analysed in this way. Child abuse in various forms has always existed; but the processes through which it is defined – and indeed what *counts* as child abuse – have changed significantly over time. During the 1980s and 1990s in particular, various concerns about 'threatened children' – from homeless children to 'crack babies' to the victims of paedophiles – came to dominate the public agenda. Children were increasingly presented as endangered and vulnerable to harm; and parents were urged to take responsibility for their protection, and for the development of a healthy personality. As Best argues, contemporary images of children as victims resonate very effectively with the idealized, sentimental image of childhood that became culturally dominant in the nineteenth century, initially among the middle class. Children themselves are also relatively low in the hierarchy of claims-makers: they are rarely consulted – for example in media or policy debates – thus leaving the way clear for adults to make claims on their behalf (Loseke, 2003).

Indeed, making children the focus of claims often provides a powerful means of pressing emotional 'buttons', and hence of commanding assent, even when the actual target is much broader. If harmful influences in society can be shown to impact specifically on children, the argument for controlling those influences comes to appear much stronger. For example, Philip Jenkins (1992) provides a detailed study of the role of claims-makers and 'moral entrepreneurs' in the moral panics around child abuse – from sexual violence to paedophilia to Satanic rituals – which became so prevalent in Britain during the 1980s. As Jenkins shows, campaigns against homosexuality were redefined as campaigns against paedophiles; campaigns against pornography became campaigns against child pornography; and campaigns against immorality and Satanism become campaigns against ritualistic child abuse. Those who had the temerity to doubt spectacular claims about the epidemic proportions of such phenomena – or to question the need for censorious or authoritarian forms of action – could thereby easily be stigmatized as hostile to children. While some of the campaigns Jenkins identifies have faded, others have replaced them, and some have become steadily more prominent: concerns about childhood have become a powerful dimension of much broader assertions about the unravelling of the social fabric, and the moral collapse of what the Conservatives call 'broken Britain'.

The point here is not that these problems are merely illusory, or just a matter of irrational panic – although that probably is the case with some of the examples analysed by Jenkins. Rather, the focus of analysis is on how the problem is socially defined and constructed, and by whom; on the assumptions and emotional responses that are invoked in the process; and on the ways in which alternative perspectives are thereby excluded. In particular, as Jenkins (1992), Sternheimer (2010) and others argue, there is a risk that the construction and framing of specific social problems may divert attention away from more complex, more intractable issues – notably those which relate to the economy, and to social deprivation and inequality.

The problem of the child consumer

To what extent might we see the 'problem' of children and consumption in these terms? In recent years, there has been a flurry of popular critical publications about children and consumer culture, following in the wake of Naomi Klein's influential *No Logo* (2001). Prominent examples include Juliet Schor's *Born to Buy: The Commercialized Child and the New Consumer Culture* (2004), Susan Linn's *Consuming Kids: The Hostile Takeover of Childhood* (2004), Alissa Quart's *Branded: The Buying and Selling of Teenagers* (2003), Daniel Acuff and Robert Reiher's *Kidnapped: How Irresponsible Marketers are Stealing the Minds of Your Children* (2005) and, in the UK, Ed Mayo and Agnes Nairn's *Consumer Kids: How Big Business is Grooming Our Children for Profit* (2009). To be sure, there are some important differences among these publications. For example, Schor's is the most academic, and presents detailed statistical evidence from a psychological study of the links between consumption and 'materialism'; while Quart's is essentially a journalistic exposé of the teen marketing industry. As 'claims-makers', the authors also speak from different positions: Mayo, for example, is the director of a consumer pressure group, while Linn is a child psychiatrist, and Acuff and Reiher are both marketing consultants. However, these books share a highly critical view of the negative influence of advertising and marketing on children's lives: they all have a strong campaigning edge, and several of them conclude with a 'manifesto' and a series of links to activist organizations.

On one level, the arguments being made here are far from new. One can look back to similar assertions about the harmful influence of advertising being made in the 1970s, for example by campaigning groups like Action for Children's Television in the United States (see Hendershot, 1998; Seiter, 1993). However, there is a new tone of urgency here: these critics argue that contemporary marketing is significantly more sophisticated, and that children are now caught up in a powerful, highly manipulative form of consumer culture that is almost impossible for them to escape or resist. They accuse advertisers and marketers of using increasingly devious and deceitful techniques in order to target children, and of flouting legal regulations on the promotion of harmful products. They argue that children are being targeted at a younger and younger age, and that the boundaries between childhood, youth and adulthood are being progressively eroded, as children increasingly gain access to sexual and violent material. According to these critics, this new commercial culture is actively opposed to children's wellbeing and their best interests.

While there are certainly truths in some of these claims, all these books link the issue of consumerism with other time-honoured concerns about media and childhood, thereby broadening the scope of the problem and creating a picture of wholesale decline. Thus, as well as turning children into premature consumers, the media are accused of promoting sex and violence, junk food, drugs, tobacco and alcohol, gender stereotypes and false moral values, as well as contributing to an 'epidemic' of mental health disorders, anxiety, stress and harmful addictions (including the addiction to consumption itself). Today's children suffer from what Linn calls 'impulsivity' or Acuff and Reiher call 'Invisible and Intangible Information Overload' (IIIO). Children's play has been devalued, and their capacity for creative experience has been destroyed, in favour of conformity and superficial, materialistic values.

Of course, this is a familiar litany, which tends to confuse very different kinds of effects and influences; and it is informed by a much wider critique of 'consumerism', which sees it as fundamentally opposed to positive moral or human values. Linn (2004), for example, describes consumerism as an attack on democracy and family values, and on 'the spiritual, humanistic, or ineffable splendors of life' (p. 185). This ties in with a broader account of social and cultural decline, which sees children as increasingly threatened and endangered. Thus, Acuff and Reiher (2005) begin their book by declaring: 'Parents, your children today are in greater physical, psychological, emotional, and ethical danger than during any other era of modern civilization' (p. xii).

Perhaps paradoxically, the most vehement of these texts is that written by the two marketing consultants, Acuff and Reiher, whose biographies boast an extensive list of high-profile corporate clients. These authors employ the full range of rhetorical strategies that are characteristic of social problems claims-makers. Parents are addressed – via the collective 'we' – as partners in a crusade. A large collection of authorities is enlisted in support, by means of short (and frequently platitudinous) quotations that scatter the text, seemingly at random, from Billy Graham and Martin Luther to Albert Einstein, James Baldwin and Eleanor Roosevelt. Scientific evidence, principally drawn from infant neuroscience ('brain science') and developmental psychology, is presented as undisputed truth. The core chapters of the book present lists of 'basic needs', 'core developmental elements' and 'key vulnerabilities' relating to children at each of Piaget's developmental stages. Yet these apparently scientific arguments about the 'wiring' of the brain and about 'developmental blind spots' are used to justify what are clearly *moral* judgements, particularly about the influence of sexual and violent content in the media – for example about 'age-inappropriate sexuality' and the promotion of 'irresponsible attitudes'.

Lurking behind these judgements are further prejudices about taste and cultural value. Commercial marketing is acceptable, it would seem, if it promotes products that are 'healthy' or 'wholesome', but not if it relates to things that the authors deem to be harmful. For each age group, Acuff and Reiher present 'a week in the life' of an ideal and a dysfunctional family, arranged in two parallel columns. While the good parents set boundaries, preserve quality time and generally promote a healthy learning environment, the bad parents are permissive and neglectful (they send their children to daycare!), and allow their own enjoyment of popular culture to act as a model for their children. The contrast here is so absolute and stereotypical as to be comical – indeed, it rather resembles a meeting between the Brady Bunch and the Bundy family from *Married with Children*. While the teenagers from the good family are at their church group meeting, listening to 'soft rock' and reading poetry, the bad ones are wearing trenchcoats and miniskirts, playing violent computer games and generally living the life of sex, drugs and gangsta rap.

Collectively, these texts tell a simple story of the struggle between good and evil. Children are represented here as essentially innocent and helpless, unable to resist the power of commercial marketing and media. They are seduced, controlled, manipulated, exploited, brainwashed, bamboozled, programmed and branded. They are seen as fundamentally passive, vulnerable and defenceless – as 'passive commercial fodder', 'cogs in a wheel' or, in the words of Acuff and Reiher, 'sitting ducks' and 'easy prey' for marketers. Yet, as with other such campaigns invoking children, these books rarely include the voices of children themselves, or try to take account of their perspectives: this is essentially a discourse generated by adults *on behalf of* children.

The marketers, meanwhile, are the original Hidden Persuaders of popular legend (and indeed Vance Packard's classic Cold War paranoia about the thought-controlling power of subliminal advertising is quoted approvingly by several of these books: Packard, 1957). Marketers are seen to be engaged in a 'war on children': they bombard, assault, barrage, and even subject them to 'saturation bombing'. They 'take children hostage', invade, violate and steal their minds, and betray their innocence and trust. Even Mayo and Nairn (2009), who tend to represent children as more sceptical and resistant to the appeals of advertising, nevertheless present marketers in highly melodramatic terms. The subtitle of their book effectively equates marketers with paedophiles, while terms such as 'grooming' and 'stalking', and the metaphor of the 'child-catcher', recur throughout (on publication, an extract from the book was published in *The Times* newspaper accompanied by a large image of the evil Robert Helpmann character from *Chitty Chitty Bang Bang*).

As the social constructionists would put it, this story resonates very powerfully with the dominant 'feeling rules' of contemporary society (Loseke, 2003). Children reside in the highest moral category: they are constructed as blameless victims, innocent and morally pure. The marketers represent their moral counterpart: they are the smug, evil villains of the piece, deserving of our most vehement condemnation.

However, the intervening role of parents here is somewhat more ambivalent and problematic. 'Good' parents – those implicitly addressed by these books – exercise proper protection and control over their children, while 'bad' parents are liberal and permissive, indulging their own and their children's consumer desires. Ultimately, parents appear strangely powerless in the face of the 'onslaught' of commercial marketing; and yet they are also somehow to blame for what is happening to their children. In this context, 'good' parents can all too easily slip into being 'bad' parents, whether as victims of ignorance or of their own lack of self-discipline. Acts of consumption – whether by children or parents themselves – require constant vigilance and supervision, ideally armed with the checklists and 'toolboxes' such publications provide. Thus, while all of these books call for some kind of ban on marketing to children, or at least for much tighter regulation, much of the onus for dealing with consumer culture ultimately falls to parents; and indeed much of the rhetoric appears designed to inflame parental anxiety and guilt. The only solution, it seems, is for parents to engage in counter-propaganda, to censor their children's use of media, or keep them locked away from corrupting commercial influences. Only then, it would seem, when their lives are wholly supervised and controlled, will children truly be free to be children once more.

Childhood at risk

As I have implied, these concerns about the influence of advertising and marketing on children are typically implicated within a broader narrative about the fate of contemporary childhood. In this narrative, modern childhood is characterized not as a period of carefree innocence, but as one of danger and risk; and, indeed, as a time of anxiety, misery and stress. While this bleak image of childhood has arguably been around for a long time, it has become much more culturally dominant in the first decade of the twenty-first century.

The most spectacular focus of this concern is of course that contemporary 'folk devil', the predatory paedophile. Despite the fact that the large majority of child abuse occurs within the family home, it is predominantly understood – not least by children themselves – as a matter of 'stranger danger'. Indeed, it would seem from some popular accounts that the paedophile is no longer lurking only in the street or in public spaces, but in your child's school or nursery, or indeed on the computer in your child's bedroom. Joel Best's (1990) analysis of moral panics surrounding 'threatened children', noted above, suggests that the contemporary rhetoric of 'child-saving' is typically justified by using melodramatic images of children menaced by deviants, in the form of paedophiles, child pornographers, kidnappers, drug pushers and Satanic abusers. To this cast of evil-doers, it would seem, can now be added the figure of the marketer as child-catcher.

This growing concern over child safety has resulted in what some commentators have seen as a culture of 'over-protection', and even of 'paranoid parenting' (Brooks, 2006; Furedi, 2008; Guldberg, 2008). Critics of such developments recount tales of schools being banned from videotaping children's Christmas plays on the grounds that the tapes might be obtained by paedophiles, or barring parents from sports events for fear that child abusers might attend.[1] At the time of writing, a group of leading children's authors in the UK has proposed to abandon readings of their work in schools if they continue to be subjected to police checks designed to identify sex criminals.[2]

However, others argue that this 'cocooning' of childhood now extends far beyond the fear of sexual abuse. At least in the UK, children are now much more confined to their homes, and much less independently mobile, than they were thirty years ago. Since the 1970s, 'playing out' in the street or in open spaces has steadily been displaced by domestic entertainment (particularly via television and computers) and – especially among more affluent classes – by supervised leisure activities such as organized sports, music lessons and so forth (Valentine, 2004). An extensive 'health and safety industry' has arisen to market 'safety-conscious' products to parents of very young children (Martens, 2005), supported both by the general climate of anxiety and by restrictive legislation. Mundane playground conflicts between children have been subjected to new forms of therapeutic intervention, and a whole range of everyday emotions (such as shyness) have been classified as psychological 'syndromes' that are in need of expert treatment (Guldberg, 2008).

As we shall see in subsequent chapters, parents are also increasingly urged to take responsibility for ensuring their children's educational success. 'Good' parenting is now seen to involve constant surveillance, in order to ensure that your children are engaged in worthwhile, self-improving learning activities; and, of course, many companies (from educational publishers and software companies to the providers of supplementary classes and home tutoring) have seen this as a lucrative commercial opportunity. Many of these arguments are also frequently justified by what might be called 'infant determinism' – the claim, apparently bolstered by evidence from neuroscience, that children's later development is heavily dependent on the growth of the brain in the early years of life.

Toxic childhood syndrome

Here again, it is possible to track the activities of some prominent 'moral entrepreneurs' involved in these debates. As we have seen, claims-makers are bound to compete with each other in the public arena in seeking to name and define their chosen social problem. Their aim is to achieve 'ownership' of the problem; although in doing so, they will often seek support from a wide range of allies – sometimes allies who are otherwise quite incompatible. And as we have seen, claims about children carry a particular weight in what Best (1990) calls 'the social problems marketplace'.

In the UK, this has been particularly apparent in the recent debate about 'toxic childhood'. Assertions about the 'loss of childhood' have a long history: Neil Postman's *The Disappearance of Childhood* (1983) is one notable example, although much older instances can be found in the literature on 'moral panics', particularly in relation to media and popular culture (Buckingham, 2000a; Springhall, 1998). However, Sue Palmer's best-selling book *Toxic Childhood: How the Modern World is Damaging Our Children and*

What We Can Do About It, published in 2006, has enjoyed remarkable success in reviving the argument, and effectively defining a contemporary 'syndrome'. The publication of the book was quickly followed by a letter that appeared in the *Daily Telegraph* in September 2006: almost certainly orchestrated by Palmer, the letter was signed by a wide range of campaigners, academics, medical experts and children's authors, and received widespread publicity.[3] The *Telegraph* immediately launched a campaign to halt the 'death of childhood', and this in turn seems to have prompted the Children's Society to undertake its 'Good Childhood Enquiry', a longer-term initiative which eventually resulted in the publication of the book *A Good Childhood: Searching for Values in a Competitive Age* (Layard and Dunn, 2009), subsequently followed by the Society's *Manifesto for a Good Childhood*.

There is an underlying religious dimension to this debate, which is implicitly signalled by the use of terms like 'values'. The Children's Society is in fact a Church of England organization, although it does not always make this explicit; and the Patron of its Enquiry was Rowan Williams, the Archbishop of Canterbury and Leader of the Church of England. Palmer's book was preceded by a number of high-profile interviews and articles in which Williams challenged what he regards as the influence of secular commercial forces in British society.[4] In political terms, the argument is somewhat harder to pin down: although the *Daily Telegraph* is certainly a right-wing newspaper, the signatories of Palmer's letter were politically quite diverse. Indeed, the ensuing debate over 'toxic childhood' was subsequently joined by publications in a similar vein from the Labour campaign group Compass (*The Commercialisation of Childhood*, 2006) and the National Union of Teachers (*Growing Up in a Material World*, 2007).

While there are some differences between these texts, Palmer has been particularly effective in establishing her 'ownership' of the problem (not least by follow-up publications such as *Detoxing Childhood: What Parents Need to Know to Raise Happy, Successful Children*, 2007). Her image of contemporary childhood, and of the modern family, is unremittingly bleak. Children, she argues, are increasingly unhappy and dissatisfied with their lives. We are apparently witnessing a mental health crisis among young people, which is manifested in rising levels of binge drinking, eating disorders, self-harm and suicide; in the increase in Attention Deficit Hyperactivity Disorder (ADHD), dyslexia and autism spectrum disorders; and more generally in increased levels of depression, anxiety and poor self-esteem. Children's relationships with others are more competitive and superficial, resulting in a growing incidence of emotional difficulties, bullying and violence; and their lifestyles are increasingly unhealthy. Children today have a poorer attention span and less ability to tolerate deferred gratification: 'every year [they] become more distractable, impulsive and self-obsessed – less able to learn, to enjoy life, to thrive socially' (Palmer, 2006: 14). There has been an erosion of respect for authority, as society has drifted into moral relativism: children are increasingly lacking in discipline, respect for others and good manners. All these symptoms, she argues, are particularly manifested among working-class children, who are 'increasingly feral' and live 'chaotic, dishevelled lives'.

Amid this catalogue of woe, Palmer identifies three fundamental causes. Firstly, and most importantly, children's increased access to media and technology – and to consumer culture more broadly – is seen to have damaging effects on their behaviour and attitudes in a whole range of areas. These include: levels of fear and anxiety; sedentary lifestyles; withdrawal and isolation; 'pester power', peer pressure and bullying; distractedness, reduced attention spans and sleep deprivation; the lack of family conversation and interaction; disrespectful behaviour and insolence towards adults; and the undermining of imagination and creative play. While Palmer condemns the internet as a forum for paedophiles, pornographers, psychopaths and terrorists, she accuses the media more broadly of promoting aggression, desensitization to suffering, sexualization, gender stereotyping, obesity, eating disorders, bad language, 'sleazy' lifestyles, bullying and materialistic values. These assertions are imbued with a familiar rhetoric about manipulation, addiction, passivity, brainwashing, bombardment, 'instant gratification' and the whole 'imagination-rotting, creativity-dumbing whirlwind' of contemporary popular culture (2006: 229).

The second cause is to do with changes in family life, and changing ideas about parenting; and in this respect, Palmer's account locks into well-established arguments about the 'crisis' of the modern family. The growing involvement of women in the workplace, the rise in divorce and single-parent families, and pressures of work apparently mean that parents spend less time with their children. On the one hand, parents no longer exercise sufficient responsibility, for example in determining what children eat, how they spend their time, when they get to bed, and so on. The 'conventional disciplinary father figure' has, according to Palmer, unfortunately disappeared. Yet on the other hand, parents are also too protective, for example in excessively supervising their children's play, or in 'hot-housing' children by filling their time with improving activities. It is not clear

Oxford Brookes University
Harcourt Hill Campus

Customer ID: ******81839

Title: material child : growing up in
consumer culture
ID: 0096427606
Due: 18 December 2015

Title: Children, adolescents, and the
media
ID: 0085795709
Due: 18 December 2015

Total items: 2
09/12/2015 15:29
Checked out: 8
Overdue: 0

Thank you for using the
3M SelfCheck™ System.

whether the neglectful, the over-indulgent and the over-authoritarian styles of parenting apply to different social groups, although there is an implicit class dimension here. Palmer offers plentiful tips for parents on 'detoxing' childhood; but they are also portrayed as relatively powerless in the face of the 'onslaught' of media and marketing.

Finally, government policy in a whole range of areas is also accused of reinforcing 'toxic childhood syndrome': over-protective health and safety legislation, the undue emphasis on testing in schools, lack of support for family life, failure to provide adequate childcare, and so on. Schools are hampered by bureaucracy, teachers are compelled to teach to the tests, children are led into formal learning too early, and there is a damaging culture of educational competitiveness both inside and outside schools. At the same time, what Palmer calls 'misinterpretations' of human rights legislation have further promoted the culture of moral relativism and 'market-driven self-indulgence'.

Of these three elements, the first is ultimately the most significant: weaknesses in the family, and failures of government policy are seen to have created a kind of moral vacuum into which the damaging influences of media and consumer culture can enter.

Modern life is rubbish?

The 'toxic childhood' position shares several characteristics with earlier campaigns of this kind, although the target of its criticism is rather more diffuse and all-encompassing. Indeed, it is hard to think of many things that are wrong with the world that do not come under its remit. Ultimately, it amounts to a comprehensive rejection of modernity – a stance that is explicit in the subtitle of Palmer's book. In this respect, it might be seen to stand in a time-honoured British tradition, which can be traced back at least to the Romantics. Modern technology, urbanization, consumer capitalism, the pressure to compete, and the 'speed' of contemporary life are the villains of the piece, while there is a strong sense of nostalgia for a simpler, slower time, a rural idyll of family togetherness and spontaneous play, in which 'children could be children'.

Indeed, the comprehensive range of its critique may partly account for its success: there is something for everyone to agree with here. As I have noted, childhood serves as a particularly powerful unifying symbol in this respect: dissenters can easily be stigmatized as uncaring and neglectful of children's needs, if not as outright enemies of childhood. The very simplicity of the story also accounts for its ability to attract publicity and command assent. It is a story that cannot be allowed to have a positive side: arguments that might imply that children have more choices, opportunities, autonomy and rights than they used to do cannot be permitted – or they can only be acknowledged if these things are seen as fundamentally misguided (as is the case in Palmer's discussion of children's rights). The causal explanation that is proposed here also needs to be kept as simple as possible. Palmer insists that the phenomena she describes are complex and have several causes – although her account of the influence of the media and consumer culture is resolutely one-dimensional, even if her view of changes in family life is rather more ambivalent. There is a kind of grandiose cultural pessimism here: the modern world is seen to have collapsed into a spiral of inexorable moral and cultural decline. Essentially, we are all going to hell, and it's the media and consumer culture that are taking us there.

Children are represented here as vulnerable victims, rather than in any way resilient or competent. The banal possibility that most children (and their parents) are reasonably well adjusted and doing fairly well – or simply that society has become more fluid and diverse – is not one that can be entertained. Palmer's (fictional) portrait of a typical contemporary child, with which her book begins and ends, is entirely negative: it is hard to imagine how such a miserable, dysfunctional being could manage to survive. There is also an implicit class bias in the arguments. Palmer consistently assumes that the problems of modern childhood are more prevalent among working-class children. It is working-class families that are almost invariably represented as the most dysfunctional; and it is among working-class children that the most challenging and socially unacceptable forms of behaviour are apparent. Palmer claims to be drawing attention to the problem of inequality, but her terrifying picture of the 'feral' children of the working classes is suffused with class-based judgements to do with taste and morality.

Of course, it is important to assess such assertions on the basis of the evidence. Much of the evidence cited here amounts to hearsay and anecdote. Scientific authorities are quoted, statistics from opinion polls are proffered, yet there is no systematic critical presentation of data. There is a persistent confusion in the argument between correlations and causes; and incompatible or contradictory phenomena are attributed to the same fundamental cause. The basis on which historical comparisons are being made is frequently unclear. I will return to these issues in detail, and present a range of contrary evidence, in later chapters. Yet questions of logic and proof seem almost beside the point in this context. Like other such 'moral entrepreneurs', Palmer speaks at a fundamentally emotional level – and, at times, at an almost visceral one. She seeks to persuade, to command assent, through the telling of a story about childhood – a story that speaks to, and mobilizes, some of the most deep-seated hopes and fears of parents in particular. The key issue, therefore, is not so much to do with whether this story is accurate, but with the emotional responses and the underlying assumptions that it invokes. Every construction of a 'social problem' involves a set of choices, a way of framing the topic, which effectively precludes other ways of seeing or understanding it. The question here is to do with what is gained – and more particularly, what is lost – in this process.

Kid power?

The image of the child consumer and the story of modern childhood I have been analysing here stand in stark contrast to the views of marketers themselves. As such, this is hardly surprising, although (as we shall see) it does result in certain paradoxes. I will be considering contemporary marketing to children in more detail in chapter 5; but it is worth elaborating briefly on this contrast here, as it illuminates some of the implicit assumptions about childhood that are at stake in this debate.

As the children's market has grown in size and influence, there has been a proliferation of marketing discourse that seeks to explore and define children's characteristics and needs as consumers. While campaigners on these issues often conceive of children as passive victims of commercial manipulation, marketers are inclined to profess a very different view. They tend to construct the child as a kind of authority figure: children (who are almost always referred to here as 'kids') are seen as active, competent and 'media savvy', and hence as extremely difficult to reach and persuade. In fact, this attempt to define and celebrate the power of the child consumer also has a fairly long history, reaching back at least to the 1920s, when retailers and advertisers began to orient themselves more directly towards children, rather than their mothers. As Dan Cook (2000) observes, market researchers have increasingly represented children as powerful, autonomous consumers: their desire for commercial products is frequently seen as a form of 'self-expression' and a manifestation of their individuality.

One contemporary example of this approach may be found in the book *Brandchild* (2003), written by the self-professed 'brand futurist' Martin Lindstrom and his colleagues. Apparently based on research with 2,000 children worldwide conducted by the advertising agency Millward Brown,

Brandchild focuses primarily on 'tweens', which it defines as children aged 8–14. The book argues that there is now a growing need for marketers to recognize and respond to the changing needs of this newly identified 'niche' market. According to Lindstrom, tweens are a digital generation, 'born with a mouse in their hands'; and they speak a new language, called Tweenspeak. They have anxieties – the stress of growing up, the fear of global conflict, and so on; yet brands can help them to enjoy life despite their difficulties. Indeed, tweens are seen to have a 'spiritual hunger', which brands and marketers alone can satisfy.

The theoretical and methodological basis of this kind of market research deserves critical scrutiny – and Lindstrom's book has come in for some scathing criticism within the market research industry (Fletcher, 2003). However, the most striking aspect in terms of our focus here is the very different construction of the child consumer. Far from being a passive victim, the child here is sophisticated, demanding and hard-to-please. Tweens, we are told, want to be in control, to be 'listened to, heard, respected and understood': they must not be patronized. Tweens, Lindstrom argues, are not easily manipulated: they are an elusive, fast-moving, even fickle market, sceptical about the claims of advertisers, and discerning when it comes to getting value for money – and understanding and capturing them requires considerable effort. As such, they are extremely powerful and influential consumers: 'they get what they want when they want it'.

Of course, that is not to say that this market cannot be persuaded or won: books like *Brandchild* are replete with suggestions for how to target (and indeed manipulate) children. Like many of their critics, the marketers often display a profound faith in the science of developmental psychology, offering detailed analyses of children's innate emotional 'needs' at different ages and stages (see also del Vecchio, 1997; Sutherland and Thompson, 2001). Significantly, the tactics that Lindstrom recommends to reach tweens, such as viral and peer-to-peer marketing, rely on the active participation of the peer group – and they are precisely those that most alarm those who campaign against consumer culture. For the marketers, however, these practices are all about empowerment – about children registering their needs, finding their voices, building their self-esteem, defining their own values and developing independence and autonomy.

The contrast between this argument and that of the critics of consumer culture creates some interesting paradoxes. The campaigners who purport to be speaking on behalf of children and defending their interests tend to present them as powerless; while the marketers, who might be seen as attempting to manipulate them, present them as powerful. The supposedly 'radical' critics of consumerism fall back on traditional constructions of children as innocent and vulnerable, passively socialized by external forces and lacking the skills or rationality adults are assumed to possess; while the marketers emphasize – and indeed celebrate – children's autonomy, competence and independent agency. Of course, marketers are bound to present children in this way, in order to deflect accusations that they are merely exploiting them. Their claims about the scepticism and sophistication of children – and indeed about the limited influence of advertising – are routinely invoked in response to public criticism. Yet such claims nonetheless bring them closer to recent thinking in the Sociology of Childhood, and in the area of children's rights, which has tended to challenge conservative views of children's innocence and vulnerability, and argued for a view of the child as a competent social agent (A. James et al., 1998).

In the highly polarized debate about children's engagement with the commercial world, this creates a paradox – and indeed a political dilemma. There seems to be a stark choice here. Do we side with the critics, who are undoubtedly identifying some significant problems in the way the market operates, but who tend to rely on a traditional, conservative view of childhood? Or do we side with the marketers, on the grounds that they appear to believe in children's power and autonomy – even as they are accused of seeking to undermine it for their own ends? In the public arena – and even, to some extent, in the academic debate – there seems to be very little possibility of finding a middle ground between these positions, or of moving beyond what seems to be a simple either/or choice.

Yet, despite their differences, these two positions also appear to construct and define childhood in similar ways. While the campaigners assume that there is a 'natural' state of childhood that has been destroyed or corrupted by commercialism, the marketers suggest that children's 'real' innate needs are somehow being acknowledged and addressed, even for the first time. It is believed that there is something particular to the condition of childhood that makes children necessarily more vulnerable — or else spontaneously more wise and sophisticated, for example in their dealings with technology; and that adults are somehow exempted from these arguments. Both approaches rest on assumptions about the natural or innate characteristics of children, which are in fact socially and historically defined. Both appear to place childhood in a space that is somehow outside or beyond the social world – and hence the commercial world as well. By contrast, I would argue that what Dan Cook (2000) calls 'commercial epistemologies' are an unavoidable part of the construction and make-up of childhood itself. Rather than the commercial world being an add-on, or an invasion of childhood, it is an inevitable part of it; and we need to pay careful attention to the ways in which those on all 'sides' of this debate construct and view children.

Conclusion

The social constructionist approach I have adopted in this chapter has undoubted limitations. In rejecting 'objectivism' – the notion that social problems simply exist out there in the world, waiting to be recognized – it runs the risk of its opposite, relativism. It has been accused of providing no basis for judging whether claims about social problems are true: all we have is a mess of claims and counter-claims, with no means of adjudicating between them (see Loseke, 2003). In practice, however, social constructionists appear to step back from this position: they remain interested in establishing the *real* scale of the social problems they address, and in identifying their empirical causes and consequences. The fact that problems are socially constructed does not mean that they do not exist; and the ways in which they are constructed also have material implications for people's lives, in terms of their access to resources and how they relate to each other.

The particular value of this approach, however, is in helping us to understand what might be gained and lost in constructing problems in particular ways and not others. The metaphor of 'framing' is especially useful here. Framing defines a problem, what is important about it and why it matters; but, in the process, it also prevents other possible definitions and explanations, and obstructs the consideration of other potentially relevant issues. The frame includes, but it also excludes. Social constructionists typically differentiate here between *diagnostic* frames – which specify the nature, meaning and cause of the problem; *motivational* ones – which explain why people should care about it; and *prognostic* ones – which identify what needs to be done (Snow and Benford, 1988). In the case of children and consumption, the construction (or the dominant critical framing) of the problem has significant limitations. I will define these in broad and general terms at this stage: specific illustrations and examples, which will undoubtedly complicate the story, will be addressed in subsequent chapters.

In terms of the *diagnostic frame*, the problem is fairly narrowly defined, as a question of children's exposure to advertising and marketing in particular: other forms of commercial or economic activity to do with the production and circulation of goods and services are much less likely to receive attention. The relationship between children and advertising (or marketing) is predominantly defined in terms of cause-and-effect – as a matter of influence that flows only in one direction. In the process, children are largely seen as passive victims, and as particularly vulnerable to influence, by virtue of their (lack of) psychological development. Furthermore, certain *kinds* of consumption – which are deemed excessive or unnecessary, or which relate to products that are deemed to be harmful or morally undesirable – are seen as problematic, while others are rarely mentioned.

In terms of the *motivational frame*, the issue is defined much more broadly. The problem of children's relationship with advertising and marketing is caught up in a much more all-encompassing story (a grand narrative) of social, cultural and moral decline. This story is one with clearly defined 'goodies' and 'baddies', in which innocent children are preyed upon and ultimately violated by evil marketers. The telling of this story inevitably connects with broader cultural themes, and invokes 'feeling rules' that make it clear to us why we should care. It draws upon long-standing sentimental views of childhood, which present children as threatened and endangered. It also invokes underlying assumptions about cultural value, reflecting a profound distaste for the unrestrained and vulgar consumption practices of those who are defined in various ways as Others.

Finally, in terms of the *prognostic frame*, there is a peculiar imbalance. Most critics call for a partial or complete ban on advertising and marketing to children; but in practice – and in the likely absence of such a ban – they tend to address their recommendations for action to parents. The problem is effectively individualized, and the responsibility for addressing it is placed on parents. Parents are strongly urged to pursue 'good' (that is, restrained, wholesome and tasteful) consumption practices, and to eschew 'bad' ones, both for themselves and on behalf of their children. Good parents are offered extensive instruction in ways of supervising and regulating their children's consumption, and thereby ensuring their healthy psychological development.

One key aim of this book is to offer some way of *reframing* the 'problem' of the child consumer. Evaluating the kinds of claims that are made about the problem is inevitably part of this: evidence about the extent of various aspects of the phenomenon, and their causes and its consequences, can and should be carefully assessed. But beyond this, I shall be suggesting some new ways of defining and understanding the issues at stake, which go beyond the current terms of the debate. To begin, in the following two chapters, this will involve exploring some of the theories and assumptions that have been entailed in academic accounts of consumer culture, both in general and then specifically in respect of children.

2

Understanding consumption

The popular debates considered thus far inevitably invoke broader assumptions both about consumption and about childhood itself. This chapter therefore takes a step back from these debates to consider more theoretical approaches to the study of consumption and consumer culture. In fact, while the tone of academic scholarship may be different, many of the basic views expressed here are very similar to those of the campaigners and the marketers considered in the previous chapter. Researchers and theorists have been quite polarized in their interpretations of consumption, although yet again the dominant view is very much a negative one. In outlining a range of academic perspectives here, one of my key aims is to suggest some ways of moving beyond this rather unproductive debate.

Children have rarely been a significant concern in academic studies of consumption, and as such they barely feature in this chapter. In chapter 3, I will seek to explain why this should be, and how the child consumer has been – and could be – understood theoretically.

Theorizing consumption: the bad news

In recent years, consumption has been an increasingly popular focus of study across a wide range of disciplines, including economics, sociology, anthropology, history, psychology and cultural studies. My account here can only hope to skim the surface of this work: there are several good introductory accounts of the field, most of which cover very similar ground, albeit with different emphases (e.g. Aldridge, 2003; Bocock, 1993; Corrigan, 1997; Edwards, 2000; Gabriel and Lang, 2006; Lury, 1996; Mackay, 1997; Miles, 1998; Paterson, 2006; Slater, 1997).

As Raymond Williams (1976) and others have noted, the earliest uses of the term 'consume' date from the late Middle Ages, and tended to be highly pejorative: to consume meant to use up, to destroy, to waste. Indeed, the word 'consumption' also originally referred to a wasting disease, and eventually became the popular term for what we now call pulmonary tuberculosis. Williams argues that the negative connotations of the term steadily faded during the nineteenth century, as the consumer emerged as a key figure in liberal economic theory. However, I would argue that the pejorative connotations of the term have never entirely disappeared. In both popular and academic debate, a view of consumption as essentially and inherently bad sits awkwardly alongside a more neutral usage. For example, the term 'consumerism' is sometimes used to describe the movement for consumer rights (particularly in the United States: see Cohen, 2003); but it is also widely used to identify a set of beliefs that are seen as fundamentally false. The ideology of consumerism, it is argued, is one in which the purchasing and possession of things is held to be more important than people, or than lasting human values.

As Aldridge (2003) suggests, this position could perhaps be seen as a vestige of Puritanism, and its moral disapproval of extravagance and self-indulgence. However, in practice it often appears that only certain kinds of consumption are judged negatively: the generalized condemnation of consumerism is often infused with distaste for the vulgar and excessive consumption practices of *other people*. And while there are frequent expressions of disdain for the 'conspicuous consumption' of the *nouveau riche* – those who aspire to join the middle class, but tend to have more money than good taste – these other people have historically always belonged to the lower orders. Thus, there is a long tradition, dating back to early debates about the harmful habit of novel-reading, of regarding *women's* consumption as somehow inherently problematic. Contemporary jokes about 'retail therapy', 'fashion victims' and 'shopaholics' are almost universally applied to women, and betray a continuing view of women's consumption as somehow excessive, trivial, irrational and even pathological – while men's consumption is, of course, implicitly defined as autonomous, self-controlled and rational. Meanwhile, rising levels of affluence among the working class (which will be considered more fully in chapter 8) have led to the emergence of another category of 'bad consumers', who are often deemed to be consuming in a manner that is unrestrained, unseemly or harmful. The problem with working-class consumers is that they obstinately insist on consuming the *wrong things*. In contemporary Britain, the consumption practices of those who are frequently derided as 'chavs' are increasingly stigmatized as lacking in restraint and good taste (Hayward and Yar, 2006). The current debate about children's consumption can also be understood in this context. As I have implied, children are easily 'othered' in this debate, perhaps particularly because they are rarely heard or consulted: children's consumption is generally constructed as a problem in a way that (some) adults' consumption is not.

These negative views of consumption (or, more specifically, of 'consumerism') are not merely popular prejudices: they are also very often implicit in the academic debate. Indeed, they form a powerful dimension of what Celia Lury (1996) calls the 'producer-led' critique of consumer culture. While it can largely be identified with the political left, elements of this argument frequently recur right across the political spectrum; and this is by no means the only possible 'left-wing' position. The argument has a long history, and many variants, but it can be fairly crudely summed up as follows.

Capitalism is an inherently unstable system, based on the exploitation of the mass of the proletariat by the ruling class. One way in which the ever-present threat of revolution can be forestalled or prevented is through deluding the proletariat into believing that the system works in their interests, or that they might have something to gain from it continuing. Mass consumption effectively achieves this, not only through the provision of affordable commodities, but also by creating a system of meanings and pleasures that motivate the purchasing and possession of goods. Particularly through the means of advertising and marketing, modern capitalism effectively creates false needs (or confuses desires with needs), which it then claims to satisfy. It encourages us to buy things we do not need, and offers us magical solutions to problems that we didn't even know we had. By misleading and manipulating people into the pursuit of material possessions, capitalism undermines authentic social relationships, replacing them with a form of competitive (and acquisitive) individualism. And yet people's true needs – for identity, community and human values – can never be met in any lasting way by the superficial pleasures of consumption; and this in turn provokes an unending, but always unfulfilled, search for happiness and satisfaction through yet more consumption. Ultimately, consumerism offers nothing more than a set of dreams – although these dreams have an extraordinary power to legitimate the social order, and to exert social control.

Proponents of this argument frequently suggest that in the last few decades Western capitalism has entered a new phase (although whether or not we choose to label this 'postmodern' is a can of worms that might best be left unopened here). In our contemporary 'post-scarcity' society, basic material needs (for example, for food and shelter) are generally met, and consumption has become largely driven by symbolic systems of meaning. People's sense of identity now derives from their roles not as workers or producers, but as consumers. Yet while consumers may be seduced into believing that they are actively defining their own wants and needs, in fact the market manipulates and regulates their desires, and thereby constrains their choice and freedom. Contemporary consumer culture offers experiences that are pre-packaged, alienated and lacking in creativity; any pleasure that may be experienced is short-lived and will never satisfy human beings' need for love and friendship, or their quest for identity and spiritual meaning.

This denunciation of consumerism self-evidently forms part of a broader critique of contemporary 'free-market' capitalism. In this account, the pervasive ideology of consumerism is both a symptom and a cause of the steady decline of civil society and public life. The citizen has been replaced by the atomized individual consumer, and the public sphere has come to be dominated by inauthentic commercial trivia and superficial promises of instant gratification. In the UK, as in many other countries, this critique is also informed by a degree of resistance to 'Americanization'. The US culture industries are seen here as purveyors of a commercially produced *mass* culture, which has been imposed upon, and ultimately destroyed, the authentic or 'organic' *popular* or *folk* culture of the working class.

Two contemporary perspectives

Needless to say, this critique of the dehumanizing power of consumerism and mass culture rarely appears in the simplistic form I have outlined here. However, more elaborated versions of the basic approach can be found throughout the history of modern social and political thought. Elements of the argument can be traced from Marx's ideas of alienation and commodity fetishism, through the arguments about 'mass deception' proposed by the Frankfurt School, to the critique of the 'one-dimensional' nature of modern capitalism developed by the New Left in the 1960s. At the same time, the argument has a good deal in common with much more conservative forms of social theory, for example in the work of defenders of 'high culture' such as F. R. Leavis and Ortega y Gasset (historical overviews and critiques of these arguments may be found in Carey (1992) and Swingewood (1977)). Although it has an overtly political or ideological motivation, this approach is also clearly suffused with cultural judgements about aesthetics and taste, and with moral judgements, for example to do with the dangers of self-indulgence and excess. It would seem that in these respects, the right and the left unite in a shared sense of disappointment at the irrational, vulgar and selfish proclivities of 'the masses'.

This baleful account of consumerism is also a continuing presence in contemporary social theories that purport to offer a more sophisticated approach. Two recent instances of this will have to suffice here. Zygmunt

Bauman is widely regarded as one of the leading modern theorists of consumption, and his book *Consuming Life* (2007) represents one of his many recent contributions on the topic. It is a relentlessly (and repetitively) pessimistic account, albeit one that rarely deigns to offer substantial empirical evidence. According to Bauman, consumption has now become central to people's lives: it is the condition of their identity, their very reason for being. The power of consumerism is apparently inescapable and all-encompassing: the state has become merely 'an executor of market sovereignty', and there appears to be no corner of human life left untouched by market forces. Bauman writes without qualification of the 'overall and comprehensive commoditization of human life' and 'the triumph of rampant individual and individualizing consumerism' (pp. 120, 145). Consumerism, he argues, neutralizes all dissent and resistance. People are trained and coerced into conformity, obeying the rules of the market while mistakenly believing that it sets them free. They are powerless to resist 'the conquest, annexation and colonization of life by the commodity market', and 'the elevation of the written and unwritten laws of the market to the rank of life precepts' (p. 62).

Yet, ultimately, this power is based on illusion and lies: it bypasses reason, and depends merely on emotion. For Bauman, consumer capitalism is a domain of false dreams and fairy tales: it promises to satisfy our needs, but it never can – not least because if it did so, people would stop spending. The market operates by stimulating and yet simultaneously frustrating desire; and as such, it offers only anxiety and misery. Consumerism destroys human sympathy, community and our sense of responsibility for others: it has led to the 'decomposition and crumbling of social bonds and communal cohesion' (p. 144), the destruction of truly intimate relationships, and the growth of political apathy. Consumers live only in the moment, endlessly seeking to replace what they have bought with yet more new products: 'the consumerist syndrome has degraded duration and elevated transience', and is premised on 'speed, excess and waste' (pp. 85–6). Consumers are overloaded with trivial information, and deluged with products that are instantly disposable. Indeed, the 'most closely guarded secret' of consumerism is that it is now beginning to turn the self into a kind of commodity: by cultivating a persistent fear of inadequacy, consumerism forces people to work to improve their market value by virtue of what they buy, and thence to 'sell' themselves in the marketplace of human relations.

My second example here, Benjamin Barber's *Consumed* (2007), is a less abstract text, but one that largely shares the view of consumerism as an all-encompassing, and indeed wholly negative, force. This is perhaps best summed up in the book's subtitle: *How Markets Corrupt Children, Infantilize Adults, and Swallow Citizens Whole*. Although Barber in fact says relatively little about children, *Consumed* does provide an interesting example of how ideas about childhood (and indeed 'infantilization') are invoked in the service of wider critiques of modern society. In this respect, it has something in common with Palmer's *Toxic Childhood* (discussed in chapter 1), even if its politics are ultimately rather different.

According to Barber, the commercially driven infantilization of modern (American) culture involves a privileging of the fast over the slow, the simple over the complex, and the easy over the difficult. These characteristics can be seen in a vast range of contemporary phenomena, from television, movies and video games to sports, eating habits, political debate, academic plagiarism and the rise in divorce (and the list goes on). In each case, Barber sees evidence of the inexorable dumbing down of consumer capitalism, the dominance of 'unadventurous puerile taste', the retreat from grown-up responsibility and the emphasis on 'self-involved personal choice and narcissistic personal gain' (2007: 15). Modern culture is portrayed as a world of 'compulsory attention deficit disorder', in which everything has become 'shallow, superficial, forgettable, meaningless' (p. 102): this is a world of inauthentic ('faux'), homogenized products, which trivialize human needs, reducing them to a demeaning, voyeuristic spectacle. Consumerism has effectively taken control of all human life, destroying social diversity, and colonizing time and space. Individuals are at the mercy of media monopolies, 'the shameless lords of the omnipresent pixels'. Consumers have become 'clones', suffering from 'compulsive shopping disorder', 'addictive materialism' and 'obsessive consumerism'. And yet, here again, it would seem that the power of the market is based merely on illusion: while offering dreams and promises of happiness, it can create only misery.

Barber attempts to distance himself from what he terms the 'hyperbole' of the old Marxist critique of mass culture, and to resist the patronizing notion of 'false consciousness'; but his vision of the 'totalizing' control of commercialism, and of the 'controlled regression' and 'nullity' of contemporary consumerism, clearly stands in the same time-honoured tradition. Unlike Bauman, Barber does see some way out in the form of anti-globalization campaigns, and his book concludes with a call to arms against the 'culture of infantilism' – although it is a call that carries strong echoes of much more conservative attempts to defend high culture.

The good news?

While this broadly pessimistic account of consumerism continues to serve as a kind of default position in a great deal of cultural theory, it has gained some additional traction in recent years through its critical engagement with an alternative, much more optimistic, approach. In the terms provided by Celia Lury (1996), this is a 'consumer-led' approach; and it is frequently identified both with cultural studies and with postmodernism, although in my view neither is an especially accurate label. The key advocate of this view was John Fiske (e.g. 1987, 1990), although other versions of the argument can be found in the work of authors such as Paul Willis (1990) and Mike Featherstone (1991).

As in the 'producer-led' approach, consumption is seen here as an inescapable and fundamental dimension of contemporary life. Yet, far from being passive dupes of the market, consumers are regarded here as active and autonomous; and commodities are seen to have multiple possible meanings, which consumers can select, use and rework for their own purposes. In appropriating the 'symbolic resources' they find in the marketplace, consumers are engaging in a productive and self-conscious process of creating an individual 'lifestyle' and constructing or 'fashioning' their identities. In the process, consumers are seen to be evading or resisting the control of what Fiske calls 'the power bloc', and in some respects to be already empowered or liberated.

Various metaphors are used here to identify this potentially political dimension of consumer behaviour. Fiske, for example, presents consumers as being engaged in a 'semiotic guerrilla war' with the producers and designers of goods, actively making their own meanings, often in ways that challenge or go beyond those that are intended. In some instances, the consumer is represented as a kind of artist, creatively appropriating and refashioning commodities in the attempt to express their own needs and desires, through a process of 'bricolage' (or 'do-it-yourself'). In other cases, the consumer is described as a cosmopolitan 'flâneur', an idle stroller in the cityscape, observing and flirting with the surface appearances of consumer culture, yet without any necessary commitment to its values. Elsewhere, following Michel de Certeau (1984), the consumer is represented as a 'poacher', trespassing on the land of the powerful, stealing their goods, employing the opportunistic tactics of the weak to contest and undermine the calculating strategies of the strong. Far from being deceived or deluded, consumers here are both knowledgeable and playful: they are active participants in what Fiske terms a 'semiotic democracy'.

To some extent, this argument can be interpreted as a reaction against the perceived Puritanism of the 'old left' critique – although it would certainly also claim to be politically progressive. Rather than regarding the pleasures of consumption as morally suspect – or indeed as a form of delusion – they are seen here as having a potentially transgressive, subversive dimension. In this account, popular consumption poses a threat to established cultural hierarchies and norms, and indeed to the 'tyranny' of rationality itself. The active play of the consumer thus comes to be seen as a form of resistance to the forces of homogenization and containment: consumption is not yet a revolutionary act, but it can certainly involve 'putting one over' on those in power.

It is interesting to note that, while it is much more recent in origin than the more pessimistic critiques considered above, it is hard to find unapologetic contemporary examples of this more optimistic approach. In some respects, the argument may have been a creature of its time. The later 1980s – when many of these accounts were published – was a period of significant soul-searching for the British left, as it sought to come to terms with the apparent success of Thatcherism in gaining support among Labour's traditional working-class constituency. There was a reluctance to regard the working class as simply the victim of a kind of ideological 'confidence trick'; and, most notably in the journal *Marxism Today*, there was a serious (albeit quite awkward) attempt to understand the appeal of the 'consumerist' values that Thatcher and her cohorts appeared to represent (e.g. Hall and Jacques, 1989). To some extent, the approach to consumer culture adopted by Fiske and Willis might be seen as a contemporary academic counterpart to this so-called 'New Times' movement.

Beyond the binaries

Academic debates about consumer culture have thus been characterized by a degree of polarization that in many respects echoes that of the popular debates considered in chapter 1. This has perhaps been particularly the case in my own field of media and cultural studies, where a great deal of heat has been expended in the stand-off between 'producer-led' and 'consumer-led' approaches. The work of Fiske, for example, met with a swelling chorus of academic disapproval in the early 1990s, much of which seems, in retrospect, unduly harsh.[1] Fiske and others were ritualistically accused of offering a merely celebratory account of consumerism, in which the necessary defence of popular culture had slid into a kind of superficial populism, which effectively undermined the grounds for 'real' political struggle. The more confrontational critics such as Jim McGuigan (1998) went so far as to align Fiske with neo-liberal economists like Margaret Thatcher's favourite, Frederick Hayek. Fiske and others were presented here as merely apologists for capitalism, promoting the neo-liberal doctrine of 'consumer sovereignty' – the idea that consumers are rational, knowledgeable agents, freely making choices in the marketplace.

This kind of polarization often entails a degree of mutual caricature. If Fiske emerges here as a simple-minded populist, joyfully engaging in semiotic subversion by wearing his ripped jeans to go window-shopping at his local mall, the likes of Bauman and Barber can certainly be painted as lugubrious cultural pessimists, or indeed 'Grumpy Old Men'.[2] This may be fun, but it is hardly conducive to serious discussion. Furthermore, this kind of polarization tends to present the debate (yet again) in terms of simple either/or choices. Either we believe in the power of consumers, or in the power of the market; either consumers are autonomous, or they are enslaved; either consumerism is the end of civilization as we know it, or it is the domain of a new 'semiotic democracy'; either we are optimists or we are pessimists; and so on. The problem here, of course, is that there may be elements of truth in both positions, and indeed that in some respects the two may not be quite as incompatible as they seem.

The two sides of this debate could be seen to represent the two sides of a very well-established tension in the human sciences much more broadly – that between structure and agency. To what extent are individuals simply the products of broader social forces and structures, such as social class or ethnicity, religious or political ideologies, or the economy? Or to what extent are they the authors of their own destinies, able to make their own choices and judgements, to determine their own values and lifestyles, and to act on their own behalf? Do we construct our world, or is our world constructed for us by forces that are outside our control? Or, to put it even more simply: where does the power lie?

This is of course a vast theoretical debate, which we cannot enter here. However, the basic implications for the study of consumption and consumer culture are self-evident. For many theorists, the problem becomes one of *balancing* the power of the economic system (structure) with the power of the individual consumer (agency). In textbook overviews of the field (such as those cited above), there is often a kind of see-saw effect here. At some points, structure is 'bracketed off', while at others agency is; and each is implicitly seen as a kind of qualification of the other. So, in some cases, we are told at length about the power of the marketers – although we are then reminded that we mustn't forget that consumers are not passive dupes. Or we are told at length about the creative ways in which consumers fashion their identities in the marketplace – and then we are reminded that consumers' agency is determined in the last instance by the goods (or meanings) that are made available to them by producers. More agency appears to mean less structure; more structure means less agency. There is a kind of 'zero sum game' here – a fixed amount of power seems to be available, and the question is how we divide it up between the participants. And so we often arrive at elegant but nevertheless rather generalized conclusions, such as that 'consumers make meanings, but not under conditions of their own choosing' (an echo of Marx himself, of course).

One problem with such debates is that they seem to presume that structure and agency are fundamentally opposed. Asserting the agency of consumers necessarily means denying the power of producers, and vice versa. In the case of media, this has sometimes led to a rather futile stand-off between 'consumer-led' and 'producer-led' approaches. There clearly is a problem with the view that consumers are simply the dupes of some all-powerful 'consciousness industry', or that their desires are merely the result of deception and manipulation by powerful forces that are beyond their control. Yet this is not necessarily to suggest that, on the contrary, consumers are wholly autonomous, free to create any and every meaning they choose. To assert that consumers are 'active' is not to imply that producers are powerless to influence them – although, equally, asserting the power of producers should not necessarily imply a view of consumers as passive dupes of ideology.

Anthony Giddens's theory of structuration (e.g. Giddens, 1984) is frequently cited here as a possible way of moving beyond this dichotomy between structure and agency. In essence, Giddens suggests that structure and agency are interrelated and mutually interdependent: agency necessarily works through structure, and structure necessarily works though agency. Each effectively requires the other. Where Giddens's work is somewhat lacking, however, is in its empirical specification of how these processes occur (see Parker, 2000). Even so, it seems reasonable to propose in principle that production and consumption are not opposed, but on the contrary two sides of the same coin. Production depends upon consumption: if there are no consumers, there is no profit to be made. Yet consumption also depends upon production: if there is no profit, there will be no commodities to be consumed. At the same time, this process is by no means seamless: vast numbers of new products are launched and marketed, which (for many reasons) consumers fail or refuse to take up, and financial profit is obviously far from guaranteed.

While this notion of structuration might be seen to offer a theoretically elegant solution, the contrast between the two positions I have outlined continues to raise some difficult, unresolved questions. Three broad areas of debate might usefully be flagged up at this point. The first is to do with the notion of *activity*. It seems hard to deny the fact that consumers are always, to some extent and in some ways, active: they make choices, they use commodities, and they make sense (or meaning) of what they do. As we consider the ever-growing range of products available on the market, it is also fair to suggest that they are doing so in increasingly diverse and individualized ways. Of course, it is possible to argue that such diversity is merely illusory – and indeed that the market operates by creating an illusion of diversity, when in fact everything is more or less the same. One could also suggest that activity itself is equally illusory – that consumers believe themselves to have some degree of autonomy, when in fact they are merely 'clones', programmed by the marketers. Ultimately, however, I do not believe that this view of consumption as a kind of dream, or a gigantic ideological confidence trick, can reasonably be sustained.

Even so, the notion of the active consumer has taken on a new, and more complex, aspect in contemporary consumer culture, not least because of the advent of more interactive media. As we shall see in greater detail in chapter 5, contemporary approaches to marketing (not least to children and young people) positively depend upon the active participation of the individual consumer – although, equally, there are significant questions about the limits and the significance of that participation. In this context, it seems especially important to emphasize that *activity* is not necessarily the same thing as *agency* (or power).

The second issue here is to do with *wants and needs* (see Campbell, 1987). The 'producer-led' approach typically assumes that consumers' authentic needs are ignored – or, alternatively, that false needs are created – by the market, while the 'consumer-led' approach seems to assume that consumers simply find and use commodities provided by the market to fulfil their pre-existing (inherent, or at least latent) needs. However, both sides of the debate seem to duck the question of how we might distinguish between wants (or desires) and needs, or between authentic needs and inauthentic ones. Sociologists typically distinguish here between 'instrumental' and 'expressive' needs, while psychologists tend to make use of Maslow's 'hierarchy of needs', in which basic needs (for example, for food and warmth) lead on to more complex needs (for security and protection), and thence to higher-order needs (for respect, self-esteem and 'self-actualization'). Yet, as Campbell (1987) suggests, these theories may well not correspond with how individuals understand and prioritize their needs; and, even more fundamentally, we might well ask where needs (or wants) come from, and why and how they change. Again, these issues are particularly pertinent to children: arguments about children's inherent needs often carry significant moral weight, and adults (especially parents) are constantly obliged to make distinctions between wants and needs on children's behalf.

Finally, there are questions about *knowledge*. As Mark Paterson (2006) puts it, the debate about consumer culture often rests on a distinction between the *savvy* consumer and the *sucker*. While the producer-led approach typically presents consumers as duped or deluded, the consumer-led approach tends to present them as knowledgeable and sceptical. From the producer-led perspective, the power of marketing and advertising is seen to operate on a fundamentally emotional level, bypassing rationality. By contrast, the consumer-led approach veers between a kind of celebration of emotion and pleasure (as somehow necessarily transgressive) and a view of consumption as a more or less deliberate and conscious process of self-determination, and even of political resistance. There are significant questions here, not only about the extent and nature of consumers' knowledge and understanding – for example, of marketing and advertising – but also about its consequences in terms of their behaviour. The debate often appears to be premised on a distinction between emotion and rationality – as though each might have the ability to overcome or liquidate the other. But can we assume that 'savvy' consumers are necessarily less amenable to persuasion? Are rational actors somehow able to resist emotional appeals, or is it possible that marketing can work on several different 'levels' at the same time? As we shall see, these issues have a particular relevance to children, who are typically believed to lack the knowledge and rationality that adults are assumed to possess, and hence to be more vulnerable to the appeals of advertisers. Each of these issues will be taken up in more detail, and in relation to different topics, in the following chapters.

Consumption as a social and cultural practice

Both the approaches I have outlined thus far appear to accept the idea that, in contemporary industrialized societies, consumption has increasingly become a *cultural* phenomenon. It is no longer simply an instrumental matter, of fulfilling basic physical needs (for food, warmth and so on). On the contrary, it is much more to do with cultural symbols and meanings: it is a matter of aesthetic taste and style – particularly, although by no means exclusively, at the level of visual appearance and design (Lury, 1996). As we have seen, it is possible to regard this as merely a matter of illusion and mystification, or, alternatively, as a domain in which consumers are active and creative participants.

However, much of this argument seems to be premised on a fundamentally individualistic view of consumption. By contrast, I would argue that consumption cannot be seen as an isolated act: on the contrary, it is inevitably embedded within everyday life and interpersonal relationships, and in wider social and cultural processes. In seeking to understand this contextual or relational aspect of consumption more fully, many researchers have adopted a broadly anthropological or sociological approach. This approach will be developed in more detail in relation to children in subsequent chapters (especially chapters 8 and 9). A brief indication of some of the key themes of this approach, and the broader issues at stake, will be offered here.

As we have seen, critics of consumerism tend to regard the cultural or symbolic dimensions of consumption as somehow irrational, or merely as a consequence of manipulation (Campbell, 1987). From this perspective, human needs are innate, while wants or desires are merely cultural – and in this case, effectively imposed by capitalism (and especially by the 'consciousness industry' of marketing and advertising). Yet anthropological studies show that consumption – the acquisition, display, use and giving of goods – always carries symbolic functions, even in pre-industrial and non-capitalist societies. Consumption is never merely instrumental: it is also always expressive. It is not just about what we need to survive and function, but also about how we communicate with others, and define and construct our identity. As such, it depends upon people learning to interpret cultural symbols, acquiring particular cultural values and following (or at least understanding) cultural norms.

Mary Douglas and Baron Isherwood (1979), in one of the founding texts in the anthropology of consumption, argue that goods should be seen as 'communicators' which make 'visible and stable the categories of culture'. Drawing on evidence from studies of tribal societies, they argue that consumption can be seen as a ritual activity, which serves particular functions in terms of classifying and attributing meaning to people and events. People's relationships with goods need to be understood not simply in terms of use value, but also in terms of public meaning: consumption is not only a matter of what we *do* with goods, but also with what they *say*. This is by no means a fixed process, but one of ongoing negotiation and redefinition; and far from being an artificial imposition of capitalism, it is a necessary condition of social life.

This anthropological approach overlaps with a sociological one. Perhaps the founding father here is Thorstein Veblen (1899/1975), whose analysis of the 'conspicuous consumption' of the emergent 'leisure class' of late nineteenth- and early twentieth-century America fed into a broader theory about the use of consumption – and particularly the public display of goods – in defining social hierarchies. Veblen's somewhat sarcastic account focuses on how the 'gentlemen of leisure' use the ostentatious display and consumption of goods to signal their social superiority, both through their own behaviour and in the 'vicarious' consumption of their wives and servants. According to Veblen, this form of ostentatious consumption provided a powerful model for those in lower social classes to emulate.

This work can be seen in some respects as an antecedent of Pierre Bourdieu's equally well-known analysis of the hierarchies of taste in 1960s France in his book *Distinction* (1979). According to Bourdieu's famous aphorism, 'taste classifies, and it classifies the classifier': through the cultivation and display of particular cultural and artistic tastes, we differentiate ourselves from others, and thereby make implicit claims about our identity and social status. Bourdieu's detailed empirical analysis maps the landscape of taste onto a social world that is seen as differentiated both by economic capital and by 'cultural capital' – in effect, the forms of expert knowledge and dispositions towards cultural matters that people acquire both through formal education and through informal social exchange. He finds consistent patterns of distribution of cultural tastes and values, and coherent clusters of associations between tastes in different fields (such as music, books and visual arts), which he broadly categorizes as 'highbrow', 'popular' and 'middlebrow'.

Both Veblen and Bourdieu have been accused by subsequent commentators of being unduly deterministic and inflexible in their analyses, although it should be pointed out that the specific societies they discuss were much less mobile, and arguably much more hierarchical, than those of contemporary Western industrialized countries. In this sense, their work can more usefully be seen as evidence of a particular historical and cultural context: the 'war of position' or the competition for social status they describe undoubtedly continues today, but it may be taking an increasingly complex and diverse form.

Thus, more recent theorists have argued that in the contemporary (and perhaps postmodern) context, social and cultural hierarchies are no longer as fixed, or indeed as singular: there are multiple, competing social hierarchies; social groups are more loosely defined; and there are no longer fixed status groups. As a result, the distinction between high culture and popular culture has become much more fluid, and there are much more diverse forms of cultural capital at stake (Bennett et al., 2009). Meanwhile, postmodernists typically argue that we have seen a proliferation of information, products and images, in which signs or symbols have become increasingly detached from their referents, and meaning is becoming significantly harder to pin down (Featherstone, 1991). This has led some to replace the notion of social class – which remains fundamental to Bourdieu's analysis – with the more flexible, or perhaps merely individualistic, concept of 'lifestyle' (Miles, 1998). The anthropologist Daniel Miller (1987) provides a rather less relativistic development of Bourdieu's approach, arguing that the consumption practices of particular social groups are no longer so coherent or consistent: rather than seeking to emulate or aspire to their social superiors, subordinate groups may create their own cultural forms and hierarchies, not least by virtue of the ways in which they appropriate consumer goods. As such, any attempt to map consumption practices onto social categories and distinctions is much more complex, although it is by no means doomed merely to describe a picture of infinite diversity.

This broad approach has been developed though a wide range of empirical studies of historical and contemporary consumption. For example, researchers have explored changes in eating and drinking practices, and how these relate to broader changes in social mores and the relations between social groups (see Corrigan, 1997: ch. 8). To be sure, questions about what, how, when and where we eat and drink are partly a matter of the 'political economy' of food production, but they also reflect consumers' active construction of a shared universe of values and meanings. Taste and appetite are not simply given, but socially constructed and learned – and as we shall see in chapter 6, this has significant implications for children's diets and the creation and marketing of 'children's foods'.

Likewise, anthropological and sociological studies of clothing and fashion also focus on how consumers use clothing to construct and define their social identity (see Corrigan, 1997: ch. 11; Edwards, 2000: ch. 7; Miles, 1998: ch. 6). While this is to some degree a matter of signalling social status, research suggests that there is no simple 'trickle down' effect here: people do not necessarily seek to mimic or emulate the clothing styles of those whom they consider to be their social superiors (in the manner proposed by Veblen). Rather, the values that are embedded and communicated via clothing are diverse and multifaceted, relating to several different aspects of social identity (gender, ethnicity, class) but also to values (such as those relating to the public display of wealth, or to sexuality) (F. Davis, 1992). Again, we shall see in chapter 7 how these issues impact on children, and particularly on beliefs about how children's dress might communicate values about sexuality, or knowledge of sexuality, that are deemed to be 'inappropriate' for their age.

More broadly, Daniel Miller has developed this anthropological approach in a series of detailed empirical studies of aspects such as shopping, and the ways in which people use and display goods in the home, both in the UK and elsewhere in the world. Miller (e.g. 1987, 1998) focuses on the enormously diverse and often idiosyncratic characteristics of local and domestic consumption practices, and the ways in which people appropriate, customize and invest meaning in everyday objects. Miller disputes the abstract either/or logic that I have identified above, arguing that consumers cannot be seen either as mindless pleasure-seekers, passively manipulated by the market, or as rational 'sovereign consumers', autonomously seeking to meet their needs. In one of his most recent books, Miller (2008) also provides a significant empirical challenge to the claim – familiar among critics of consumerism – that capitalism has led to a situation where objects are more highly valued than people. On the contrary, he argues that possessions are embedded within complex networks of personal relationships, and that people who value objects also appear to value their relationships with people more highly.

It is important to emphasize that, while consumption is seen here as an active process, it is not regarded purely as a matter of individual free choice. On the contrary, it is seen as a social and interpersonal phenomenon, which is about the shared construction of social practices and social mores – about how we learn to act and the relationships we have with each other. The political consequences of this process are by no means guaranteed: it is not a matter either of manipulation by all-powerful marketers or of resistance in the manner of Fiske's 'semiotic guerrilla warfare', but rather of a complex, ongoing social negotiation, whose outcomes cannot be predicted in advance. Nor, on the other hand, are such researchers concerned to make moral judgements about whether consumption is in itself a good or a bad thing (see Miller, 1997). To this extent, this approach seems to provide a productive alternative both to the very abstract ways in which the political dimensions of consumption are typically addressed, and to the moralistic terms in which children's consumption in particular is generally framed.

Beyond consumption

Despite the many differences between the 'pessimistic' and 'optimistic' accounts of consumption, there is a shared assumption here about the importance of consumption itself, and to some extent about its essentially *symbolic* functions. Few authors on either side of the debate express much doubt about the absolute centrality of consumption, or of market relations, to modern life; and, however they may ultimately view it, few appear to question the idea that the power and significance of consumption today lie not so much in the satisfaction of material needs, or in the more 'instrumental' aspects of consumption, but rather in the realm of meaning, and even of aesthetics and 'style'. Yet some objections need to be raised on both these points.

Colin L. Williams (2005) provides an interesting challenge to the broader narrative of 'commodification' – the argument that the market is steadily and inexorably penetrating every last area of social life, and that this will only increase. Williams's particular focus is not primarily on consumption but on work. He provides a considerable body of evidence to show that, in most modern industrialized countries, 'non-commodified' work is a widespread and growing phenomenon. Included in this category are various forms of subsistence work (such as housework of various kinds), which people do in order to maintain their everyday existence; non-monetized exchange, whereby people informally undertake work or support tasks for each other without money changing hands; as well as more formal volunteer work, community-based activities and the 'not-for-profit' sector. Williams also points to various forms of resistance to commodified work and forms of exchange, and to changing attitudes towards 'work–life balance'. Interestingly, he argues that it is higher-income groups (who at least have the means to be more 'consumerist') who are increasingly undertaking such non-monetized work; and they are doing so out of choice rather than necessity, on the grounds that it is inherently pleasurable or because it provides opportunities to socialize. Williams argues that these phenomena have largely been ignored by critics of commodification, and indeed that, if anything, they point towards a growing process of *de*commodification among so-called 'consumer societies'.

Conrad Lodziak's *The Myth of Consumerism* (2002) provides a different challenge to the 'culturalist' emphasis of many contemporary analyses of consumerism. In some respects, Lodziak belongs with the 'producer-led' critics of consumer culture; and much of his book engages in a virile diatribe against what can only be called a caricature of a 'cultural studies' approach. Even so, Lodziak usefully points to the danger of focusing on the symbolic or textual dimensions of consumer culture – its signs and meanings – while neglecting the material dimensions of consumption. He argues that such an approach ignores the everyday experiences of the majority of people, even in Western 'consumer societies', in favour of those of a small elite. For most people, he argues, the bulk of consumer spending is actually on necessities; and the costs of basic survival, even in the wealthiest countries, are actually increasing. The rising price of everyday necessities, planned or accelerated obsolescence, the privatization of public services, and the casualization of labour all mean that it is becoming harder for most people to meet basic needs. As such, the 'freedom' that is allegedly available in consumer society is far from equally available to all.

Lodziak also suggests that (what he calls) 'cultural studies' significantly overstates the significance of consumption in terms of identity. Most consumption, he argues, is not expressive but instrumental – just as, for most people, shopping is not an act of semiotic guerrilla warfare, but a mundane and tiresome chore. In the process, he argues that the celebration of consumer autonomy has led to a blurring of wants and needs, and this has meant abandoning any grounds for making normative judgements about the effects of the market economy (for example, in terms of waste and pollution). In fact, he suggests, most people's needs in terms of identity formation relate to non-material factors: by contrast, the consumption of material goods relates only to relatively trivial or superficial aspects of identity (such as 'style').

In different ways, both Williams and Lodziak challenge some of the basic assumptions that characterize both 'sides' of the debate about consumer culture. They argue that a great many aspects of people's everyday lives are not in fact mediated through or organized around consumption or market relations (however broadly defined), let alone determined by them. They also challenge the notion – which appears to be taken for granted by most, if not all, the accounts I have discussed – that consumerism is in fact 'triumphant' (as Bauman would have it). And they imply that, far from being dupes of the 'ideology of consumerism' – or indeed joyful exponents of it – people may be aware of it, and seek to resist it, or at least find value in other areas of life. People may be consumers, and may have no option but to consume, but that does not necessarily imply that they are consume*rist*.

In fact, several of these points find support among the other work considered here. Miller's studies of shopping (e.g. 1998) confirm that most people's experiences of shopping are instrumental and mundane: shopping rarely carries much personal significance, let alone the level of quasi-artistic creativity or political challenge that is proclaimed by some. Even so, shopping is often a site for working through broader moral and social dilemmas. For example, although people occasionally indulge themselves in 'treats' or 'luxuries', they frequently seek to economize on their own behalf while simultaneously saving to buy gifts for other family members (particularly children). Yet, for most people, most of the time, shopping is far from being an experience of unalloyed freedom and pleasure, and merely one of functional routine.

Indeed, the 'postmodernist' celebration of the empowered, hedonistic consumer – the consumer as artist or 'flâneur' – could be seen to apply only to a relatively small proportion of the population. Of course, window-shopping at the mall is, at least in principle, free to everyone – although it is often far from easy for children and young people who are the regular targets of suspicion and harassment from security guards. Yet beyond this, few people have the extensive financial means that would be required to play in the postmodern world of free-floating signifiers – or indeed to be the 'shopaholics' or 'compulsive consumers' condemned by the critics of consumerism. At most, such images would seem to apply only to a relatively small fraction of the cosmopolitan middle class – and perhaps primarily to the 'cultural intermediaries' whom Bourdieu (1979) identifies: those working in the media, design and cultural industries who are themselves the primary ideologues of postmodernism (see Featherstone, 1991).

Indeed, it is important to remind ourselves that, even in apparently affluent, developed societies, levels of participation in consumption are very unequal. In the UK, as in many other countries, the gap between rich and poor is widening; and even though child poverty has reduced, around one third of children still live in conditions of poverty (see chapter 8). Despite some of the problems with his broader argument, Zygmunt Bauman (2007) is correct to identify the 'underclass' as the primary casualties of consumerism. Those who are unable to 'buy in' to the consumer society are typically seen as 'flawed consumers', who are only to blame for their situation: even if they are targeted by what Bauman calls 'market seduction', they are frequently unable to act on their desires. As we shall see in more detail in chapters 8 and 9, there is particular pressure on less wealthy families in this respect: poor families have to develop complex strategies for coping with the apparent demands of a consumer society, and this may be a particular issue for parents who seek to buy their children high-status goods as a means of reducing the stigma of poverty. As Edwards (2000: 129) suggests, the most significant form of oppression in relation to consumerism is not the pressure on the wealthy to spend, but the exclusion of those who are denied participation; and this in turn may well undermine feelings of self-worth, increase social isolation, and result in a growing perception of relative poverty. Indeed, it is part of the inevitable 'logic' of the market that consumers with more money to spend will be better served than those with less; and, as such, the market seems bound to accentuate inequalities. This issue of inequality will be a recurring theme in later chapters, and will be a particular focus of the final three.

Conclusion

This chapter has offered something of a whistle-stop tour of theories of consumption. There are four conclusions that I would draw at this point, which will be carried over into the account of children and consumption in the chapters that follow. These can be very briefly stated as follows:

1 The debate about consumption and consumer culture has generally been quite polarized. Moralistic condemnations of the dehumanizing effects of consumerism, and celebratory accounts of the power and autonomy of consumers, are both frequently overstated. We need to move beyond such binary, either/or choices.

2 Consumption is embedded within people's everyday lives and social relationships. It has functions that are both material and cultural (or instrumental and expressive). The consumption – purchasing, display, use and circulation – of commodities reflects broader processes of social communication and identity construction.

3 Consumption – or market relationships more broadly – is not necessarily as 'triumphant' or all-encompassing as some of its critics (or indeed its advocates) suggest. Most consumption is not a matter of obsessive compulsion, or of joyous self-expression, but rather a mundane and inescapable necessity.

4 However, a market system tends to serve most effectively those who are in a position to buy, and is bound to operate in their interests. As such, it may accentuate both the perception of inequality, and inequality itself.

As Dan Cook (2008) has amply demonstrated, children have been conspicuous by their absence from these broad-ranging theories of consumption, and from a good deal of the empirical research as well. It may be that children can be implicitly subsumed within a general theory. However, in the public debate about children and consumption, it is notable that children are routinely and often urgently singled out as a special case: as essentially different from adults, with different needs and vulnerabilities, and hence as requiring different forms of provision and intervention. These issues are considered in the following chapter, as I move on to consider some of the ways in which the child consumer has been – and in future might be – theoretically understood.

3

The making of consumers

Theory and research on children's consumption

What happens when we insert the figure of the child into these broader analyses of consumer culture? In their book *The Unmanageable Consumer*, Yiannis Gabriel and Tim Lang (2006) discuss what they call the various 'faces' of the modern consumer: the consumer as chooser, as communicator, as identity-seeker, as hedonist, as rebel, and so on. Like most analysts of consumer culture, Gabriel and Lang barely consider children – although, significantly, they do discuss youth. Yet, of all the 'faces' they discuss, it is notable that the one that applies above all to children is that of the *consumer as victim*. Like the rest of their book, Gabriel and Lang's discussion of victimhood is concerned with adults – with their experience of being ripped off and defrauded, and the extent to which they could and should be protected under consumer law. Along with Aldridge (2003), they suggest that this view of the consumer no longer enjoys the high profile it once did. But when we consider the public debate about children and consumption – and when we consider much of the research – it is clear that children are a striking exception to this. The child consumer is predominantly defined not as a rational chooser, a purposeful identity-seeker or a free-floating hedonist, but on the contrary as manipulated, exploited and victimized.

Indeed, the moralistic tone that characterizes many broader condemnations of consumer culture takes on a particular force when it comes to children. The contrast with *youth* is particularly notable here. Overviews of consumer culture typically discuss 'youth culture' as an instance of the creative autonomy of modern consumers: while recognizing that youth is a significant target market, they regard young people very much (in Gabriel and Lang's terms) as identity-seekers, rebels and artists – and on occasion as activists (see, for example, Lury, 1996; Willis, 1990). By contrast, children continue to be perceived as fundamentally without agency. They are seen to lack the knowledge and experience that would enable them to make informed choices in their own right. Their identity is incomplete, and is being formed *for* them rather than *by* them. Although they do possess needs, they are deemed to be incapable of articulating those needs, or of distinguishing them from wants. It is adults who possess the means to act; and it is up to them to act on children's behalf. It is for these reasons that children's access to the world of consumption is regarded as essentially illegitimate: it appears to be part of the condition of being a child that one should not be a consumer. And this in turn explains the complex feelings – of guilt, of responsibility, and yet also of displaced adult pleasure and desire – that are so frequently invoked when the figure of the child consumer is discussed.

Children as economic agents

This view of the child consumer might be seen to reflect a wider incompatibility between the idea of childhood and the world of the economy. Such a view is also apparent in debates about children working. The notion that childhood should be a period of play and learning, and not of work, is of course a relatively recent one. As the historian Ludmilla Jordanova has shown, criticisms of child labour in the late nineteenth century – and campaigns to eradicate it – reflected much wider beliefs about the essential nature of childhood:

> Children were [seen as] tender, impressionable, vulnerable, pure, deserving of parental protection, and hence all too easily corrupted by the market-place. Two main justifications existed for this characterisation of children: a Christian one, which portrayed children as in a 'sacred state of life'; and an ideological one, according to which they were somehow 'naturally' incompatible with the world of commodities. (Jordanova, 1989: 20)

As Jordanova argues, children's relationship with the economy is a key site of tension in their apparent transition from the status of child (in the domain of nature) to that of adult (in the domain of culture).

Contemporary discussions of children's work often reflect similar assumptions – although they are also frequently tied up with criticisms of *other* cultures in which the failure to segregate children from the world of work is seen as evidence of a fundamental lack of 'civilization'. And yet, even in Western industrialized nations, significant numbers of children continue to work in exchange for money. This is, of course, well known when it comes to teenagers, although the scope and diversity of teenagers' work goes well beyond the stereotypes of newspaper delivery, babysitting and weekend shop work (see McKechnie et al., 2004; Mizen et al., 1999).

In the UK today, the majority of older children engage in part-time paid work at some stage. Although the large majority do so for less than six hours a week, one quarter of 15-year-olds work more than this.

Furthermore, as Viviana Zelizer (2002) suggests, children under the legal age of employment are also actively involved in a whole series of 'informal' economic practices, of production, distribution and exchange. These range from involvement in family businesses, caring for family and relatives, and household work or 'chores' in exchange for cash allowances, through to systems of exchange within the peer group, for instance via gift-giving and trading of goods. In doing so, children develop complex economic relations with members of their own households, with their friends and peers, and with a whole range of other organizations including companies, shops, schools and voluntary groups. And yet, as Zelizer argues, this 'huge undersea continent' of children's productive work has largely been ignored by researchers.

Meanwhile, studies of childhood in developing countries have increasingly challenged the view of child labour as a wholly corrupting force (indeed, the use of the term 'labour' itself conveys something of this moral disapproval). While not ignoring the forms of inequality and exploitation that are often at stake here, they suggest that children's work can be seen as a key dimension of their involvement in community and family life (Katz, 2004; Nieuwenhuys, 1996). Similar arguments have been made about children's work in industrialized countries. Research suggests that paid employment can have value for young people in terms of developing self-esteem and a sense of responsibility, as well as in the development of more specific vocationally relevant skills – although it is undoubtedly the case that many employers are failing in their legal duty to safeguard children (McKechnie et al., 2004).

My focus here is on children as consumers, not as workers – although, as we shall see in more detail in chapter 5, at least part of their ability to consume clearly depends upon their ability to earn money from paid work. Yet in both respects, there is a widespread assumption that children are – or *should be* – kept apart from the economic or commercial world. Children may engage in their own 'work' of play and learning (Alanen, 2001), but they cannot be considered as active or productive economic agents in their own right. As a result, Zelizer suggests, most of the questions we ask about these matters are framed by adult concerns: they are about 'how children understand the adult economy, how they learn [about] it, how they fit in and how it affects them' (Zelizer, 2002: 377).

Psychology and the child consumer: effects studies

These latter points are certainly true of mainstream psychological and social-psychological research on children and consumption. Since the 1970s, there has been a growing body of work in this area. Much of it focuses on children's responses to advertising – especially television advertising – rather than on other aspects of marketing or of consumption. A great deal is also concerned with purchasing behaviour (or aspects of 'pre-purchasing' such as information-seeking, preference and choice); and relatively little with how children appropriate and use products in their everyday lives. As such, this work focuses on a relatively narrow aspect of the broader nexus of production, distribution, circulation and consumption. This book does not seek to provide a review of this research: such reviews can usefully be found elsewhere (e.g. Gunter et al., 2005; Gunter and Furnham, 1998; McNeal, 2007). I will be referring to some of this work in specific areas in later chapters (especially chapters 6 and 7); my concern here is with the underlying theoretical or philosophical assumptions that inform it.

Broadly speaking, childhood has been subject to a particular division of labour within the human sciences. The study of children is typically the province of psychology: although there is a burgeoning sociology of childhood (of which more below), children often do not appear to become of interest to sociologists and theorists of consumption until they pass the threshold of 'youth'. As objects of psychological inquiry, children also tend to be perceived and defined in particular ways here. The primary interest is in *internal* mental processes of cognition or emotion: the social context is predominantly understood as an external variable or influence. Children are also conceptualized principally in terms of *development* – that is, in terms of their progression towards the goal of adult maturity. And methodologically, much of the focus is on what children *think* – or say they think, often in response to psychometric tests – rather than on what they *do*, or even on how their knowledge is used in everyday life. By and large, children are not seen here as independent social actors: as sociologists of childhood would have it, they are seen not as *beings*, but only as *becomings* (cf. Lee, 2001).

In terms of the study of children and consumption, this has been manifested in two main areas of research: effects studies, focusing principally on advertising; and studies of 'consumer socialization'. Effects research remains the dominant perspective in psychological studies of children and media, and has been widely debated elsewhere, especially in relation to the topic of media violence (for recent critical reviews, see Buckingham et al., 2007; Freedman, 2002; Millwood Hargrave and Livingstone, 2006). I will consider some of this work, in relation to debates about consumption and childhood obesity, sexualization and materialism, in later chapters. Nevertheless, a few general observations should be made here about how this kind of research typically conceptualizes the child consumer.

While positive effects might in principle be acknowledged, in practice the focus of such research is almost exclusively on negative or harmful effects. In the case of consumption, these harmful effects are potentially legion: researchers have explored whether exposure to advertising and marketing results in physical and psychological illnesses (from obesity and eating disorders to anxiety and depression), the consumption of harmful products (such as tobacco, alcohol and 'junk food'), and a range of anti-social behaviours and attitudes (from materialism to conflict within the family to violence). The dominant concerns of effects research thus clearly reflect the arguments of the critics discussed in chapter 1; and the visibility of popular campaigns on these issues undoubtedly accounts – at least in part – for the extensive funding of this type of research by governments and private foundations of various kinds.

This research tends to work with a broadly positivist approach. It generates hypotheses about the social world that are then tested empirically through the application of scientific or mathematical methods, and thereby verified or falsified. It is assumed that we can measure the inherent messages or meanings of media content quantitatively; that we can do the same with audience responses; and that we can then correlate these in order to gain some measure of media effects. Potential variables in the process can be isolated and controlled, or accounted for statistically; and any potential influence of the scientist on the design or interpretation of the study can be eliminated or minimized. These approaches claim to provide predictability, objectivity and a basis for generalization; and the findings of such research can be statistically aggregated by a technique known as meta-analysis.

However, critics frequently question the validity of the methods that are used in effects research. The key problem with laboratory experiments is their artificiality: children are typically exposed to unrepresentative 'stimuli' in unusual conditions, and their resulting behaviour or attitudes are measured in artificial or unreliable ways. At best, laboratory experiments can be seen as an indication of what might possibly happen, rather than as evidence of what actually does happen, in real life. Meanwhile, questionnaire surveys rely on people self-reporting their behaviour (or hypothetical behaviour); and a great deal of such research tends to confuse correlations or associations between variables with causal relationships. For example, it is possible to show that children who watch a lot of television advertising also profess to hold materialistic attitudes. But this does not in itself prove that television *causes* those attitudes: it might equally be the case that people who are predisposed towards materialistic attitudes tend to seek out television as a form of entertainment, or indeed that there are other factors (such as social class or family background) that explain both types of behaviour. (This issue is discussed in more detail in chapter 9.)

The more fundamental objection, however, is to do with the notion of 'effect' itself. Effects research is self-evidently premised on a view of children's relationship with media as a matter of cause and effect. A classic behaviourist perspective (which is sometimes misleadingly termed 'social learning theory') conceives of this process in terms of stimulus and response – of which the most obvious example would be imitation. From this perspective, television advertising would be seen to produce direct effects on viewers – not only in terms of purchasing behaviour, but also in terms of attitudes and values. More sophisticated exponents of this approach posit the existence of 'intervening variables' (both individual differences and social factors) that come between the stimulus and the response, and thereby mediate any potential effects – although the basic 'cause-and-effect' model continues to apply. This kind of research implicitly conceives of the child consumer as a *tabula rasa* – a blank slate on which marketers inscribe their harmful messages.

As such, critics of effects research argue that it sanctions simplistic and misleading responses to complex social problems. Rather than looking at a particular social phenomenon such as violence and then seeking to explain it, effects research starts with media and then seeks to trace evidence of their harmful effects on individuals. In this respect, it appears to be asking the questions the wrong way round. Andrea Millwood Hargrave and Sonia Livingstone (2006) put this very effectively:

> Society does not ask, for example, whether parents have 'an effect' on their children or whether friends are positive or negative in their effects. Yet it persistently asks (and expects researchers to ask) such questions of the media, as if a single answer could be forthcoming. Nor, when it has shown that parents do have an influence on children, do we conclude that this implies children are passive 'cultural dopes', or that parental influence is

to be understood as a 'hypodermic syringe', as [is] so often stated of media effects. Nor, on the other hand, when research shows that parental influence can be harmful to children, do we jump to the conclusion that children should be brought up without parents; rather, we seek to mediate or, on occasion, to regulate. (p. 47)

As this implies, a more holistic account of the role of the media – and of marketing and advertising – in children's lives would enable us to move beyond simplistic ideas of effects – although it would not necessarily remove any grounds for intervention, or indeed for regulation. Criticisms of effects research do not in any way imply that media have *no* effects on people, as is sometimes alleged. Rather, they suggest that the notion of cause-and-effect is itself a narrow and misleading way of conceiving of the role of social and cultural factors (and of media) in children's lives.

Consumer socialization and its limits

While effects research is primarily based on a form of behaviourism, research on consumer socialization draws largely on developmental psychology. Here again, there is a substantial body of research – although curiously much of it dates back to the 1970s, despite the significant growth in the children's market that has occurred since that time. Extensive reviews of the findings of this work may be found elsewhere (e.g. Ekstrom, 2006; John, 1999; McNeal, 2007); here again, my intention at this point is merely to identify some of the general ways in which it defines or conceptualizes the child consumer.

Socialization is a somewhat broad concept, although it is predominantly conceived in functionalist terms: that is, it is a question of how children learn to think and behave according to dominant social expectations, and thereby become competent members of society. In relation to consumption, socialization is therefore about learning to be an effective consumer: as Scott Ward (1974) defines it, in one of the founding statements of research in this field, the term 'consumer socialization' refers to 'the processes by which young people acquire skills, knowledge, and attitudes relevant to their functioning as consumers in the marketplace'. In terms of learning, consumer socialization is thus typically seen as a progression from ignorance to knowledge, or from incompetence to competence. Here again, the child is seen very much as a becoming rather than a being; and children are defined in terms of what they cannot do, or fail to do, rather than what they can do. The social and cultural aspects of the child's experience are implicitly seen as extraneous to the process of cognitive development: the child is somehow pre-social, needing to be finished off or completed before it enters society. As with effects studies, this is often tied up with a positivist approach to research method: researchers begin with fixed notions of the competence, skills or knowledge that children need to learn (and which adults are believed to possess), and then proceed to measure the extent to which children have acquired them.

In exploring consumer socialization, most researchers have drawn on frameworks from developmental psychology in proposing a sequence of 'ages and stages' in maturation (John, 1999; McNeal, 2007). From this perspective, children's development as consumers is related to the development of more general cognitive skills and capacities, such as the ability to process information, to understand others' perspectives, to think and reflect in more abstract ways, and to take account of multiple factors that might be in play in decision-making. Influenced by parents and peers, as well as media and marketing, children's consumer behaviour is seen to become gradually more autonomous, consistent and rational. As they get older, they also draw on a greater range of information sources in making purchasing decisions. In all these respects, the period between the ages of seven and eleven years is often seen as a particularly important phase in development.

For example, this research suggests that children's identification and knowledge of commercial brands, and their consumer preferences, develop from a very young age. Children as young as two can recognize familiar packages, logos and licensed characters, and by the age of nine are as familiar with brands and associated slogans as their parents. They gradually use a wider range of perceptual cues to differentiate brands and categories of products, and make judgements about them. Very young children start to develop consistent preferences, for example for branded items above generic alternatives, and these become stronger and more sophisticated over time. Children's understanding of the symbolic significance of material goods also develops with age: as they get older, children come to understand how goods are used, for example to signal social status or group membership. Research suggests that by the age of about seven, children also start to draw inferences about other people based on the products they use, and subsequently (by the age of eleven or twelve) also on the basis of brands. Over time, brands not only come to function as perceptual cues (distinguishing one product from another), but are invested with symbolic meanings, which can influence children's self-concept and their judgements about others – although it should be emphasized that this is seen as a dynamic and interactive process (John, 1999).

There are numerous criticisms that might be made of this approach, many of which echo those made above in respect of effects research. The 'ages and stages' approach to child development associated with Piaget has been widely challenged in recent years, and in many areas (such as education) has been largely displaced by a 'socio-cultural' approach to psychology. However, it remains alive and well here, and indeed in psychological research on children and media more broadly. The danger here is partly that a mechanical 'ages and stages' approach tends to lead to unhelpful generalizations about children's capacities (or lack of them) at particular ages. However, it also results in an approach to socialization that is fundamentally teleological: it regards development as a linear progression towards the final achievement of adult rationality. Thus, as they develop, children are described as steadily 'improving', becoming 'more sophisticated' and 'more flexible', and moving from a 'limited repertoire' to a 'full repertoire' of skills and knowledge in areas such as shopping and decision-making (see Cook, 2010). Critics argue that this leads to a neglect of the ways in which children understand, interpret and act upon their world, in favour of a view of them simply in terms of what they lack. In common with developmental psychology more broadly, this approach also suffers from a neglect of the emotional and symbolic aspects of consumer behaviour, in favour of cognitive or intellectual ones.

Karin Ekstrom (2006) is one of several critics who point to the need for a more socio-cultural account of consumer socialization. She argues that consumer socialization is an ongoing, lifelong process, rather than something that is effectively concluded at the point of entry to adulthood; that it varies among different social and cultural groups, and over time; and that it involves different life experiences and contexts of consumption. As such, there can be no single definition of what counts as a 'competent' consumer. Ekstrom also argues that children should be seen as active participants in the process of socialization, not as passive recipients of external influences; and she notes that children may well 'socialise' their parents (and indeed their grandparents), for example in areas such as the use of media technology or the environmental aspects of consumption (a process known as 'reverse socialization'). As this implies, children's and parents' consumer roles are not fixed, but subject to an ongoing process of negotiation and dialogue, not least as children grow older and family structures change (for example in the event of divorce: see Collins and Janning, 2010).

Dan Cook (2010) goes further in his criticisms, arguing that consumer socialization research suffers from a limited view both of childhood and of consumption. For example, as he notes, commercial influences are often equated here simply with advertising – which is to neglect the ways in which many aspects of social and cultural life are implicated in market relations, well beyond exposure to advertising. Cook proposes that the notion of socialization should be replaced by the notion of 'enculturation', which he suggests would help to move beyond the normative, monolithic approach of consumer socialization research. He argues that children are already implicated in consumer culture from before the point of birth; and that rather than seeking to assess children's knowledge in the abstract, we need to consider how that knowledge is used (or not used) in everyday social practice. Learning to consume is seen here not as a matter of one-way transmission from parent to child, but on the contrary as a process of negotiation involving diverse social agents, in which multiple meanings are in play.

Rethinking advertising literacy

These criticisms suggest some different ways of thinking about the traditional concerns of consumer socialization research, and indeed of effects research. For example, there have been numerous studies of children's understanding of the persuasive intentions of advertising – that is, the knowledge that advertising is designed to encourage them to buy, rather than simply a neutral matter of providing information (e.g. Lawlor and Prothero, 2003; Oates et al., 2002; Young, 1990). Most psychological researchers agree that children learn to distinguish between television advertisements and programmes at a fairly early age (around three or four). Some research claims that children can identify persuasive intent by the age of around seven, although other studies suggest that, while this knowledge may be available or understood in principle, it is not necessarily always used, at least until the age of eleven or twelve – a distinction that psychologists typically define in terms of the difference between competence and performance.

Here again, there is a tendency for researchers to work with a fairly antiquated account of child development, which defines the child in terms of a deficit model. For example, the American Psychological Association (APA) Task Force on Advertising and Children (American Psychological Association, 2004) quite baldly claims that young children do not understand others' beliefs, desires and motivations, and hence cannot comprehend the nature of persuasion. As Basham et al. (2006) suggest, such a view is strikingly at odds with most of the child development literature of the past two decades; yet even if it were true, it would not necessarily follow from this that younger children are therefore more vulnerable to influence, as the APA report suggests.

In fact, when it comes to the *effects* of advertising, there is considerable doubt about whether children's developing understanding of advertising actually helps to reduce its effects. Some researchers suggest that if children do not understand the idea of persuasive communication, they are unable to use 'cognitive defences' against it – for example, by questioning the credibility of the source, or arguing against it. Some argue that children who recognize adverts as persuasive are therefore less likely to trust them, and to want the products advertised. However, this apparently commonsense assumption is not consistently supported by the evidence. It is not necessarily the case that older children (or indeed adults) are less influenced than younger children, nor that higher levels of understanding lead to a reduction in media effects (Livingstone and Helsper, 2006). We might presume that adults have a firm grasp not only of persuasive intent but also of the specific strategies that advertisers tend to use, but we cannot therefore assume that they are not influenced by advertising. Knowledge, in this sense, might not necessarily imply power.

Psychologists have sought to resolve this issue by suggesting that advertising (like other forms of persuasive communication) works in different ways in different contexts – and that it can operate at an emotional level, as well as a rational one (e.g. Fine and Nairn, 2008). In addition, it is likely that commercial messages targeting older children will use more complex persuasive techniques, which make greater cognitive demands, or which operate in a less explicit way. It has also been suggested that, as a result of their level of emotional development, older children may be amenable to different kinds of commercial appeals from those that address younger ones: some argue that teenagers have more disposable income and freedom to spend than younger children, but have yet to achieve an 'adult' level of impulse control, and may therefore be vulnerable in different ways. These suggestions remain somewhat hypothetical: relatively little research has explored them in any detail. Even so, they do imply that the psychological notion of 'advertising literacy' as a kind of rational defence mechanism, or a means of controlling one's emotional responses to advertising, would seem to be misguided (Buckingham, 1993a).

An alternative, socio-cultural account would suggest that knowledge of this kind is not simply acquired, developed and applied in the abstract. Children (like adults) may know in principle that advertising intends to persuade, but they may not necessarily mobilize this knowledge in specific real-world situations, or use it as a guide to consumer behaviour more generally. There are also a great many factors that can intervene between one's desire for a product (for example as prompted by advertising) and one's action in buying it or requesting it. In seeking to explore this question more fully, we would need a more in-depth understanding of how the meanings of commercial messages are interpreted and used in everyday social settings, and how those messages 'play out' relative to other aspects of children's social and material circumstances. Such an approach is bound to undermine the developmental assumption that there is a 'magic age' at which children are somehow fully and consistently aware of persuasive intent. It would also point to an analysis of 'advertising literacy' (or 'media literacy' more broadly) not as a set of psychological skills that live in people's heads, but rather as a phenomenon that is necessarily embedded within particular social contexts and forms of social action (Buckingham, 1993a).

Finally, it should be emphasized that these criticisms of the developmental approach should not be taken to imply that development as such is a meaningless concept: that would clearly be absurd. In most respects, children do self-evidently have less knowledge and experience than most adults; and they gradually learn about consumption as they get older – although adults continue to do the same. What is in question here is the psychological notion that learning (or development) is primarily a matter of internal cognitive functioning, and that it is an individualistic, a-social process. The implication of my argument is that we need to conceive of children not only as psychological becomings, who are to be assessed in terms of adult norms, but also as social beings in the here and now.

Making space for children in theories of consumer culture

These criticisms obviously point to the need for a more socio-cultural analysis of the child consumer. Yet, as I have suggested, sociological accounts of consumption and consumer culture have largely ignored children. Indeed, Dan Cook (2008) takes theorists of consumer culture to task on precisely these grounds, arguing that children are at best a 'minimal presence' in almost all the key texts in the field. For the most part, he asserts, children are seen as afterthoughts, 'conceptual props' or mere 'recipients of culture', rather than economic agents or consumers in their own right. The child, insofar as it is considered at all, is seen to exist outside the world of commerce, only to be brought into it by the socialising forces of parents, media and marketers. More sociological or cultural studies of children and consumption do, of course, exist, but there has been little recognition of this work within mainstream social and cultural theory. According to Cook, this reflects a wider neglect and marginalization both of children and of women – or, more particularly perhaps, of women's role as *mothers*. The rational adult male of mainstream economic theory, 'economic man', is implicitly seen as the norm.

As such, Cook argues, children cannot simply be appended to existing theories of consumption: on the contrary, some aspects of those theories may need to be reconsidered. Unlike 'economic man', children cannot be seen in individualistic terms, since their consumption is unavoidably embedded within networks of social relationships with carers and peers. Bringing children into the mix will necessarily mean taking account of the 'relational and co-productive nature of acquiring, having and displaying things' (p. 222). We will need to move beyond the notion of the consumer as an isolated individual, and individualistic notions of desire, identity and lifestyle, to focus instead on relationships and reciprocity. Furthermore, as Cook suggests, children do not stand still: they are constantly changing (and indeed developing). Challenging the teleological narrative of child development necessarily also means disputing the idea that adult consumers are fully formed, fully rational, competent actors.

Certainly, there is a current of argument within sociological accounts of consumption that continues to judge children's consumption in adult terms, and obstinately refuses to recognize its legitimacy. As with the generalized criticisms of consumer culture discussed in chapter 2, there has often been an uneasy alignment here between apparently radical condemnations of capitalism and much more conservative views, both of cultural value and of childhood itself. Critics such as Stephen Kline (1993), for example, claim that the market is inherently and inevitably inimical to the true interests and needs of children:

> The marketplace will never inspire children with high ideals or positive images of the personality, provide stories which help them to adjust to life's tribulations or promote play activities that are most help to their maturation. Business interests trying to maximize profits cannot be expected to worry about cultural values or social objectives beyond the consumerist cultural vector that underwrites commercial media. (p. 350)

Such arguments invoke all sorts of assumptions about the needs of children, and how they are to be met. Kline asserts that children require 'high ideals' and 'positive images of the personality', and that they need help to 'adjust' and 'mature' – and he implies that such things can only be provided for them by well-meaning adults, who are somehow free from commercial motivations. Childhood – like culture – is typically defined here as a pure, Eden-like space, a source of positive moral and aesthetic values, of 'imagination' and 'innocence', which is progressively invaded and corrupted by the dread hand of commerce. In the process, Kline argues, the traditional 'healthy' activities and experiences of childhood have been destroyed or replaced by superficial commercial substitutes.

As in a great deal of neo-Marxist cultural critique, Kline paradoxically takes the position of the 'old' bourgeoisie in his attack on what he sees as the new ruling ethos. For example, his contrast between the 'Golden Age' of children's literature and the limitations of contemporary children's television is suffused with value judgements that are neither explained nor justified: children's cartoons in particular are easily and comprehensively condemned as mindless, repetitive, inane and formulaic. As is frequently the case in such arguments, the analysis of cultural texts (such as toys or television programmes), or of their relations of production, is implicitly seen as a sufficient basis for assertions about their effects on audiences (in this case, children). Kline repeatedly asserts that the commercial cultural industries exert a powerful 'hold' over children's imaginations; that they undermine their capacities for critical thought; and that they routinely manipulate, deceive and intimidate children into submission. Yet he fails to support these claims about the mesmeric control exercised by consumer culture with any meaningful evidence of children's own perspectives.

As Ellen Seiter (1993) suggests, such criticisms often reflect an implicit snobbery, which is based on unarticulated middle-class (and, to a lesser extent, male) cultural values. She suggests that the critics of commercial media culture have implicitly enforced middle-class norms of 'proper parenting', and thereby encouraged a sense of guilt in those who fail or refuse to conform to them. She sees this as part of a wider process whereby male critics have condemned women for their interest in consumer goods, while assuming that they themselves are somehow not implicated in consumer culture. Such critics typically erect a distinction between 'good' consumption, which reflects refinement and restraint, and 'bad' consumption, which does not – and children's consumption is always defined here as irredeemably bad.

By contrast, Seiter argues that children's media culture may provide a space in which they can be free from the constraints and the surveillance of adults – albeit a space that is itself created by adults (that is, media corporations). The 'grossness' and brashness of many children's cartoons – not to mention the explicit subversion of some forms of adult authority

– may explicitly mark them out as a space that is 'off limits' to adults. A similar point might be made in relation to the complex and arcane worlds created by phenomena like Pokémon (see chapter 5) or by many computer games – although here it is the lack of knowledge that is required in order to participate that effectively excludes adults. As Seiter argues, this apparently 'subversive' appeal of children's culture has been around for centuries, and is certainly evident in a good deal of children's literature (see Lurie, 1990).

Critical accounts of children's consumer culture rarely consider the possibility that children's tastes might necessarily be different from those of adults. For example, it is possible that children of a certain age may actively prefer – and indeed, even *need* – stories that represent the world in terms of binary oppositions between good and bad, or which directly mock or subvert adult authority, in ways that adults might deem to be impossibly crude or stereotypical. Children may need texts such as cartoons, whose relentless energy, visual boldness and simplicity, and general lack of restraint lead many adults (and not just middle-class adults) to find them aesthetically repellent and vulgar (see H. Davies et al., 2000). Ultimately, these are issues that will not be resolved merely by appealing to unsubstantiated adult judgements of taste and cultural value, or to sentimental adult views of childhood: children's own perspectives and practices need to be much more fully taken into account.

Towards a cultural sociology of the child consumer

We might expect to find more useful evidence of children's experiences of consumer culture in the new sociological research on childhood that has emerged over the past two decades. Many of the following chapters will draw on this kind of research; but it should be noted at the outset that the sociology of childhood has also tended to ignore children's role as consumers. Here too, there seems to be a lingering nostalgia for a 'natural', pre-technological or pre-commercial childhood, and an underlying suspicion of what are seen to be inauthentic commercial impositions on children. Sociologists generally appear more comfortable discussing youth as consumers than they are considering children; and in many of the key founding texts of the sociology of childhood, the consuming child again seems to be largely an absence or an afterthought (e.g. Corsaro, 1997; A. James and Prout, 1990; A. James et al., 1998).

Lydia Martens, Dale Southerton and Sue Scott (2004) make a useful series of proposals for bringing children and parents more fully into the sociology and anthropology of consumption. While they agree that there is a need for continuing attention to the *production* of children's consumer culture, they argue that research should be focusing much more on practices of consumption, and how they fit into children's everyday lives. As they suggest, there are many ways in which existing work on consumption – including several of the theories and approaches discussed in chapter 2 – might be extended to incorporate children. For example, they show how Bourdieu's analysis of cultural capital might be applied to the study of how children learn to consume, and how 'skills related to competent practice, cultural values and the formation of taste are transmitted between generations' (p. 164). This approach might also be used to analyse how consumer goods are used to create and sustain hierarchies among the peer group – although in the process, Bourdieu's analysis might need to be extended to take account of more dynamic and 'informal' modes of transmission (see chapter 9). Likewise, they suggest that the anthropological approach developed by authors such as Daniel Miller might be extended to consider how children appropriate, personalize and recontextualize goods, not least through play, and thereby create new norms and conventions relating to material culture.

Significantly, Martens and her colleagues place a central emphasis on the role of parents: they argue that research needs to take account of the ways in which parents invest social and symbolic status in their children, and actively cultivate particular dispositions towards consumption. Parents, they argue, are typically held responsible for the competency and appropriateness of their children's consumption, acting as gatekeepers and primary facilitators of purchasing – although this typically involves a process of negotiation and bargaining. On the other hand, being a parent also entails a constraint on parents' own consumer practices, and their ability to create desirable (or even 'postmodern') consumer lifestyles and identities. As we shall see in more detail in chapter 8, there are interesting questions here about how children's consumption fits into the changing power relationships of the modern family. Parents may often be caught in an 'ideological dilemma' – on the one hand, seeking to regulate their children's consumption and hence ensure their own status as 'good' parents, while on the other seeking to encourage children's consumption as a vehicle for their own emotional investments in childhood.

A further theme in theories of consumer culture that might usefully be extended to children is that of *identity* – although here again, there may be a need to rethink some of the individualistic and normative assumptions about identity that often characterize such theories. Sociologists of childhood have proposed that the construction of childhood identities – and indeed the wider 'generational order' – is an ongoing process, in which children themselves are active participants (A. James, 1993). Leena Alanen's (2001) term 'generationing' implies that the relations between generations – and hence what it means to be a child – are defined in variable ways in the context of specific institutional and social practices (the school, the family, the peer group, as well as the market). To put this another way, we could propose that (like gender) childhood and adulthood identities are *performed* in different ways in different contexts and for different purposes (cf. Butler, 1990).

As we shall see in more detail in chapters 4 and 5, the market provides certain definitions or accounts of what it means to be a child, or a child of a certain age, or a boy or a girl; and these definitions are among the things that children use in constructing their own sense of self-identity. There are potentially multiple definitions (or narratives or images) here, which may well conflict with each other; and children may not necessarily recognize themselves in the definitions that seem to be targeted at them or allotted to them – or indeed if they do, they may well choose to reject or resist them. The market has historically functioned by creating age-based distinctions and gradations; and this process continues, for instance in the contemporary construction of the category of the 'tween'. However, these constructions are neither monolithic nor irresistible: there is an ongoing negotiation here, which in the case of tweens is most notable – and indeed most controversial – in relation to the issue of sexuality (discussed in chapter 7).

Furthermore, 'marketized' constructions of childhood identity relate to other constructions on the part of teachers or parents – if only because it is often parents who buy things for children, or give them the money they use to buy things for themselves, and (in some cases) attempt to influence how they spend it. As we shall see, market definitions are then cut across with definitions to do with ideologies of 'good' parenting, childrearing or pedagogy. Such ideologies also offer more or less influential definitions of what it means to be a child (or a learner), and indeed what it might mean to 'grow up'. Just as children negotiate with marketized definitions, so too do parents and teachers – and all of them have some power to determine what those constructions will look like. Children therefore 'perform' as children (or as children of particular ages, genders and so on) in a situation where the market offers several potential definitions of childhood identities, alongside other definitions that derive from the home, the peer group, the school, and so on.

Barbro Johansson (2010) develops a similar approach, using ideas from Actor Network Theory and from the work of Gilles Deleuze. Theoretically, this approach entails a shift from looking at social life in terms of self-contained individuals towards an emphasis on connections, networks and flows. Agency is seen here, not as a possession of the individual, but rather as something that is exercised in specific situations and events, and via 'assemblages' of human and non-human actors (including objects, artefacts and texts, as well as people). Johansson argues that this approach provides a way of looking beyond the familiar polarization between the views of children either as 'becomings' or as 'beings': on the contrary, she argues, there are elements of being and becoming in every situation. In her interviews with children, she identifies some of the different 'consumer subjectivities' that children assume: the child who saves for the future, the child who delegates choice and responsibility to parents, the child who shops, the child who collects, the child who consumes moderately and rationally, the child who influences family consumption. Yet rather than being fixed positions taken up by individual children, these subjectivities are seen as 'situational performances' that vary depending upon the context. Children may choose different, or multiple, roles for themselves, depending upon which aspects are important in different situations.

While Johansson's analysis is developed in relation to children, it clearly can apply to adults as well; and, to extend the argument, we can say that both children and adults are always both beings and becomings (cf. Lee, 2001). To return to our starting point, it might be suggested that people assume different 'faces' as consumers depending upon the social situations they encounter (cf. Gabriel and Lang, 2006). This is clearly not a straightforward matter of free choice: the market (along with other institutions) both produces and constrains the consumer subjectivities that it is possible to assume. Yet our performances or actions as consumers are also subject to a degree of choice and control on our part. To this extent, the identity – or rather the multiple identities – of the child consumer are not simply a creation of the market, but also identities that children themselves are actively constructing and performing in their everyday lives.

The child consumer: a cultural studies approach

Further theoretical and methodological resources for such an approach can be found in the area of cultural studies. Research in this field typically conceives of the relations between structure and agency by means of the 'circuit of culture' (see Buckingham, 2008a; du Gay et al., 1997). In his early influential account of this approach, Richard Johnson (1985/6) argues that culture is a social process, and that we can identify a series of 'moments' in that process which can usefully be isolated for analysis. The moment of *production* is that in which cultural objects or texts are brought into being; these *texts* take specific forms, that can be analysed in their own right; the meanings of these texts are then actualized in the moment of *reading*; and readings subsequently feed into what Johnson terms *lived cultures*, which then in turn impact back on the process of production. Social conditions and relations impinge on this process at each point. For example, production is not seen here merely as an individual 'creative' activity, but as one that is subject to specific institutional, social and economic conditions. Likewise, reading is not seen as a self-contained encounter between the individual reader and the text: on the contrary, it too occurs in a particular social context, which partly influences which readings are likely to be made. These broader social conditions do not wholly determine particular acts of production or of reading; however, they do set constraints and create possibilities which systematically favour the generation of particular meanings rather than others.

One study that illustrates the benefits of such a multifaceted approach to consumption can be found in the work of Rachel Russell and Melissa Tyler (2002). Russell and Tyler focus on Girl Heaven, a chain of UK shops aimed at 'tween' girls, offering inexpensive cosmetics, accessories and 'makeovers'. Russell and Tyler's work involves, firstly, an analysis of the *political economy* of Girl Heaven, and the perspectives of its producers, through interviews and encounters with the founding directors. Here they note how commercial marketing rhetoric draws on 'post-feminist' notions of 'girl power', and in some ways has the potential to shift the traditional values of girl culture: even if its ultimate aim is to realize economic value, it cannot be considered a wholly conservative force, as some of its critics assume.

Secondly, the authors conducted a *textual analysis* of Girl Heaven – where the 'texts' included marketing, online and promotional material as well as the shop itself, whose layout, lighting, displays and so on combine to convey the 'meaning' of 'girl' and 'heaven'. Their analysis focuses on how the shop conflates leisure and consumption and acts as a site for the celebratory 'performance' of femininity and for the realization of girls' 'dreams'. It is also constructed as somewhere mothers could come with daughters – an approach which distinguishes Girl Heaven from other commercial marketing to children, which often claims to be 'on the side of the kids' against, rather than with, their parents. This provides an interesting instance of how generational transitions and relationships (and the anxieties that surround both) may be commodified.

Finally, turning to the *consumers*, Russell and Tyler studied a group of eight 10- to 11-year-old girls, who were taken on a store visit, given money they could spend there and interviewed afterwards. Their analysis aims to convey a sense of young people as active social agents, whilst also revealing the social context – or the structural factors – within which they shape their 'becoming'. The process of becoming an adult (woman) is shaped by the existence of commercial opportunities through which it can be expressed. As this implies – and as I have argued – consumption does not stand apart, as an 'add-on' to childhood, but is deeply bound up with it. There is a complicated relationship here between consumer culture and 'doing' childhood – which, as these authors emphasize, also means doing femininity (or masculinity) at different ages. These girls were followed up two years later (Russell and Tyler, 2005), and in their subsequent work, the authors draw particular attention to the process of 'bricolage', of 'do-it-yourself' assembly, that is involved in the process of building identities.

This multifaceted approach, which is characteristic of cultural studies, therefore appears to move beyond the simple polarization between structure and agency. From this perspective, the market is seen to provide potentially multiple definitions or accounts of what it means to be a girl, which can permit elements of self-expression and symbolic creativity. This contrasts with earlier feminist analyses, which have often seen consumption solely as a site of exploitation and manipulation for women. Girl Heaven, by its very emphasis on the 'performance' and artificiality of femininity, might be said to open up a space for playing with the codes of femininity rather than adopting them wholesale. Yet, at the same time, Russell and Tyler point to the elements of conformity or constraint involved, and conclude pessimistically that the 'rigid roles on display' in Girl Heaven should caution against recent feminist thinking that has tried to reclaim the pleasures of feminine identity play. Crucially, however, they also show that young girls themselves were reflexive and aware of their ambivalent relationship with commercial culture – another aspect that critics of children's consumption tend to overlook.

Conclusion

This chapter has reviewed various ways of understanding and studying the child consumer. Here again, much of the discussion has been relatively abstract; although many of the general issues raised here will be explored

in more concrete ways in the chapters that follow. As in the previous
chapter, I have argued that we need to look beyond polarized views of
children's relationship with the commercial market: children are neither
the helpless victims imagined by many campaigners, nor the autonomous,
'savvy' consumers celebrated by marketers. We need to understand
consumption not as a matter of the dyadic relation between the marketer
and the child, but as something that is embedded within children's everyday
lives, including their relationships with parents and peers. Consumption is
not only about the marketing, advertising and purchasing of goods, but
also about how they are appropriated and used. It is by no means an all-
determining, irresistible force, whose 'effects' on individual children can
be isolated and assessed. Nor are children simply consumers 'in the making',
developing cognitive skills that we hope will equip them for adult life.
Children are always already consumers – although they are by no means
only consumers. Rather, childhood identities – including the various
identities of the child consumer – are actively constructed, not only by the
market but also by children themselves.

4

Histories of children's consumption

Commercial marketing to children is by no means a new phenomenon. On the contrary, it needs to be seen as part of the historical development of a modern consumer society – a development that can be traced back over at least two centuries. Here again, we need to understand children's consumption in the context of wider changes in the economy and in social life, particularly in the institution of the family. This chapter offers a broad summary of these historical developments. It begins with a brief discussion of the emergence of modern consumerism, and then moves on to review a range of historical accounts specifically relating to children.

The development of modern consumerism

The emergence of mass consumerism is often taken to be a relatively recent development. Popular accounts of the kind reviewed in chapter 1 tend to trace it back to the 'consumer boom' in the decades that followed the Second World War. Yet, as Don Slater (1997) reminds us, consumer culture has a long history. While consumption itself is not confined to capitalist societies, the rise of a *consumer society* – that is, of a social system dominated by the production and consumption of commodities – needs to be understood as a key part of the longer-term historical evolution of capitalism. Slater neatly tracks the idea of consumerism backwards through history, starting from the bullish assertions of the Gordon Gekko character in the 1980s movie *Wall Street*, whose famous motto 'greed is good' appeared to sum up the materialistic yuppie ethos of the time. Slater identifies similar apparent resurgences of consumerism in the 1950s, in the more conformist, suburban 'affluent society' identified by the economist J. K. Galbraith (1958); in the 1920s, with the rise of the Fordist system of mass production and the expansion of advertising; and in the mid-Victorian period, with its spectacular celebration of modern technology, for example in the Great Exhibition of 1851.

Slater argues that the origins of the consumer society can in fact be traced back to the growth of trade and global markets in the sixteenth century, an account that is supported by several historical studies. For instance, Grant McCracken (1988) points to the consumer boom in late sixteenth-century England that followed Queen Elizabeth's insistence on the nobles attending her court and participating in its ostentatious display of wealth. In this situation, the novelty of fashion came to be valued above the signs of age (or 'patina') that were apparent on family heirlooms. While these processes were primarily confined to élites, Neil McKendrick et al. (1982) point to the emergence of a more widely distributed form of consumerism in late eighteenth-century England, as members of other social classes began seeking to emulate the tastes of the nobility. At this point, they argue, modern mass consumption began to emerge, accompanied by advertising and marketing, of which the Staffordshire potter Josiah Wedgewood was a particularly successful exponent.

Slater (1997) argues that these developments reached a form of maturity in the late eighteenth century, when commercial infrastructures (of transportation, retailing and communication) led to a flood of new commodities targeted at middle-class consumers. As Colin Campbell (1987) argues, the industrial revolution of the late eighteenth and early nineteenth centuries was not merely a shift in the mode of production, but also a revolution in consumption. This was particularly apparent among the middle classes, whose growing demand for luxury goods and enthusiasm for leisure eventually began to trickle down to lower social strata. Campbell aligns the new 'consumer ethic' with the individualism of the Romantic movement, and with what he terms 'modern hedonism' – a view of life as an never-ending attempt to realize imaginative longings and fantasies through the acquisition of material goods.

These accounts have been much debated (see particularly Fine (2002) and Slater (1997)); but the central point – that consumerism is bound up with the longer-term development of modern capitalism, and not merely an invention of the past sixty years or so – is hard to refute. What remains more contentious are the political and philosophical consequences of these developments – and here we return to some of the broader arguments considered in chapter 2. In these accounts, the rise of a consumer society is typically connected with a decline in traditional forms of authority and social stratification, and with the rise of individualism – initially among the middle classes, but eventually among the population at large. It is also seen to entail a new emphasis on the cultural or symbolic meanings of goods (as embodied in aspects of aesthetics and design), rather than merely on their functionality or use value. According to Slater (1997), for example, a consumer society is one in which freedom comes to be identified with the private sphere: the influence of established forms of hierarchy has weakened, and there is a growing emphasis on individual choice. Consumption, he asserts, becomes 'the privileged medium for negotiating identity and status within a post-traditional society' (p. 29), and this is also symptomatic of 'the increasing importance of culture in the modern exercise of power' (p. 31).

While Slater, Campbell and others argue that these latter tendencies are long-standing aspects of capitalism, some commentators see them as particularly characteristic of the new phase of 'late modern' or 'postmodern' capitalism that has emerged in the past three or four decades – although the chronology here is often fairly vague. In some accounts, this new phase is explained primarily in terms of changes in the mode of production: it is part of the shift from a 'Fordist' to a 'post-Fordist' (or an 'industrial' to a 'post-industrial') system – or at least from an economy dominated by manufacturing to one dominated by service industries. Yet here again, this shift is typically connected with much broader changes both in social life and in individual identity (see, for example, Bauman, 2007; Bocock, 1993; Featherstone, 1991). Thus, it is argued that consumption has increasingly come to be seen as a more defining characteristic of individual identity than work, or indeed one's relation to the mode of production (that is, social class). In this context, the formation of identity has become a much more fluid, provisional process. Fixed hierarchies and status groups are no longer so clearly defined, and values such as deference and formality are steadily disappearing. Meanwhile, the cultural dimensions of consumption – of signs and symbols, and of aesthetics and 'style' – have become vastly more significant.

There is clearly room for debate about whether these apparently 'postmodern' developments are in fact new. Even so, it is hard to deny that there have been many significant historical changes in consumer culture in the past half-century (see Gabriel and Lang, 2006). At least in Western industrialized countries, generally rising levels of affluence, greater geographical and social mobility, and the growth of media and communications technologies have transformed everyday consumption. A significantly higher proportion of people's income is now spent on discretionary 'luxuries', and on services and entertainment, and less on 'necessities'. Advertising, packaging and branding have become increasingly important in defining the symbolic values of goods; and commercial influences have become more and more significant in areas of public life (such as education) that used to be seen in essentially non-commercial terms. Broadly speaking, we have moved from a society based on thrift and savings to one based on credit. The relations between buyers and sellers have become more impersonal, and intermediaries (such as retailers or shopkeepers) are much less significant. Consumers are addressed as active participants, with the power to choose and shape their individual lifestyles and identities; and consumption is increasingly governed by fashion, which changes at an ever-accelerating rate. Of course, there are significant dangers here, both in how we 'historicize' change, and in drawing distinctions between past and present, but it is important when we consider children as consumers not to lose sight of this broader context.

The emergence of the child consumer

Needless to say, children are rarely mentioned in these broader historical accounts: they remain largely 'hidden from history'. Nevertheless, there have been some significant historical analyses of children's consumption published in the past decade or so, which begin to make good some of the absences here. As I shall indicate, these studies also raise important questions – for example about the relations between parents and children, about the targeting of the children's market, and about the use of particular marketing techniques – that are still extremely relevant today.

The large-scale production of goods specifically for children – such as books, toys and games – can be traced back to the eighteenth century (Plumb, 1982), although instructional primers, playthings and clothes for the children of the nobility and the wealthy bourgeoisie were certainly being produced in the sixteenth century (Luke, 1989; McKendrick et al., 1982). The development of a children's consumer culture gathered pace in the mid nineteenth century, in parallel with the emergence of new, post-Romantic ideas of childhood. Just as children were being recognized as a distinct and special group – as pure and innocent, and in need of careful protection – they were also coming to be seen as a potential market.

Dennis Denisoff and his colleagues (2008) explore two key aspects of this new market: the commodification of images of children for consumption by adults; and the marketing of goods that were seen to preserve the unique character of childhood, and to confer educational value. As this implies, the principal purchasers of these goods were not children but adults – although children of all social classes were certainly exposed to new marketing techniques, such as the increasingly lavish displays of goods in product exhibitions, department stores and toy emporia. Denisoff argues that adults used both types of goods to maintain a kind of vicarious or nostalgic connection with their own childhoods.

Paradoxically, commodified representations of children (for example in periodicals and children's books) provided a kind of moral or spiritual counterbalance to the concerns that were raised by the growing pursuit of material wealth within the wider society. The aestheticized, sentimentalized image of the middle-class child was often tied up with the glorification of the family home as a feminine domain that stood outside the grubby world of labour and the economy (Kooistra, 2008). Yet, at the same time, there was growing concern about the production of cheap, inappropriate amusements targeted at working-class children, such as the sensational crime novels known as 'penny dreadfuls' and the entertainment on offer in 'penny gaff' theatres and music halls (see also Springhall, 1998): such products were seen to expose children prematurely to undesirable aspects of adult life, and thence to exert a corrupting influence on adults as well. Thus, while consumer culture was becoming a significant vehicle for adults' pleasurable investments in a particular conception of childhood, it was also a domain in which adults began to experience growing concerns about a loss of authority and control.

Parental ambivalence, toys and play

This issue of parents' ambivalence towards children's consumption is a recurring theme in the history. The sentimentalized representation of childhood innocence that was popular among the Victorian middle classes became much more widespread in the early twentieth century. This both reflected and reinforced the move to segregate children from the workplace, and from aspects of adult life and the commercial world more generally. As Viviana Zelizer (1985) describes, the economic value that children possessed as workers was gradually replaced by a new emotional value: the economically 'worthless' child became the morally 'priceless' child, to be coddled and cherished. Children were seen as emotional assets, whose role was to serve the psychological needs of adults; and adults looked to childhood – and indeed their own 'inner child' – as a source of timeless moral and personal truths. Yet for all its apparent resistance to commercialism, this new emotional investment in children – or at least in a particular *idea* of childhood – was wide open to market forces. Children were withdrawn from the corrupting influence of work, yet the market increasingly began to engage them as consumers. Pampering children with consumer goods was represented as a fundamental expression of parents' love and empathy. Such motivations were reflected in children's literature, in popular images of children (not least in the increasingly visual medium of advertising), and in the growing market for fantasy toys.

Yet as Lisa Jacobson (2004) shows, the expansion of the children's market that occurred in the United States in the early decades of the twentieth century was also accompanied by an increasing anxiety about its potentially corrupting influence on the young. Children's enthusiastic expression of their consumer desires appeared to challenge nineteenth-century ideas of thrift and self-control, and the sentimental view of children as innocent and pure; and in the process, children's consumption became the focus of much broader fears about social change, moral decline and the collapse of social hierarchy. This led in turn to concerted efforts to regulate children's consumption, and thereby to raise responsible and respectable consumers – not least through organized forms of saving and consumer training (see also Ringel, 2008).

At the same time, the growth of child psychology and its popularization in consumer advice literature led to a new self-consciousness about parenting. Play came to be seen as a form of educational work that was essential to children's cognitive, emotional and physical development (see Seiter, 1993). Parents were also urged to adopt more egalitarian approaches to child rearing; and as the average size of families fell, the value of children's play became central to the new 'companionate' ideal of family life that was widely disseminated in the 1920s and 1930s. Play was seen as a means of reinvigorating family relationships, and thereby of ensuring the emotional wellbeing of both children and parents.

In this context, children's consumption was increasingly linked to positive values of freedom, self-expression and family togetherness. As Jacobson (2004) describes, parents were urged both by child psychologists and by advertisers to equip separate playrooms with specially selected furniture and stimulating educational toys that would enable them to become playmates with their children. The playroom was at once a pedagogic space, a space where children (as 'becomings') would be prepared for adulthood, and yet it was also a space for self-expression, and for indulging children's consumer desires (as 'beings'). Significantly, the playroom was sold to middle-class parents as a healthy alternative to the dangers of public amusements: it was identified with a kind of anti-consumerism, a resistance to the debasing influence of commercial entertainment – and yet, as a costly venture in its own right, it was of course highly commodified, as well as being something that parents had to 'sell' to their children.

Gary Cross (1997) also explores this theme of parental ambivalence in his history of the US toy industry. As Cross indicates, toys were originally amusements for adults, and only came to be associated with children in the nineteenth century. The late nineteenth and early twentieth centuries saw the rise of toy marketing, in shop displays, catalogues and advertisements, although this was still mostly targeted at parents. Toys were often invested with parental nostalgia, and a notion of childhood as a period of timeless innocence, reflecting the sentimental 'valorization' of childhood identified by Zelizer (1985). Meanwhile, the emergence and popularization of child psychology led to a growing emphasis on the educational dimensions of toys: at least for the status-conscious middle classes, toys were represented as essential apparatus for children's development, and domestic play was regarded as an alternative to the 'rowdyism of street society'.

However, across the mid twentieth century, marketers gradually began to address children directly – an approach that accelerated significantly with the coming of television; and the parent was increasingly relegated to the role of 'an onlooker rather than an active participant' in their children's consumption (Cross, 1997: 10). As the toy market became more competitive and profit-driven, the focus of marketing shifted away from adult nostalgia and claims about the educational merits of play, and towards a more wholehearted emphasis on escapism and pleasure. As Ellen Seiter (1993) suggests, the marketing of toys *to parents* often continues to emphasize educational claims about the value of play – and perhaps increasingly so; but marketing directly to children typically focuses on what she calls the 'utopian impulse' of children's consumer culture – the promise of freedom from adult seriousness, authority and goal-directedness.

As such, Cross (1997) suggests, toys have played a profoundly ambivalent role. On the one hand, they have served as a vehicle for parents' hopes and aspirations: they have been celebrated not only for their educational value, as a means of training children for adult life, but also as a domain for children's freedom and imagination. Yet on the other hand, they have also increasingly become a focus of fears and anxieties about economic exploitation, declining cultural values and false ideologies. As parents have gradually been written out of the marketing equation, they have frequently come to blame toymakers for the broader problems they face in disciplining children – for promoting violence, gender stereotyping and materialism.

Cross explores similar tensions in his later work on images of children in advertising and popular media (Cross, 2004). On the one hand, children have been represented here as simple, innocent and joyful: they are depicted as 'cute' objects of parental affection, and even of worship, who need to be kept sheltered and protected from the corrupting influence of the adult world. Yet on the other hand, they have increasingly been celebrated for their autonomy and self-expression; and the impish, naughty child of the early twentieth century has steadily been succeeded by the defiant, rebellious 'cool kid' of the contemporary era. Cross argues that both these impulses have been commodified, in the sense that they both motivate adult spending on children: products are sold on their appeal to adult fantasies of the 'wondrous innocence' of childhood, *and* because they allow us a vicarious experience of childish subversion and resistance to authority. Yet the latter leads in turn to concerns about the harmful influence of consumer culture, and to attempts to regulate it – although, as Cross suggests, the boundaries of what is acceptable are constantly shifting, and adults seem increasingly uncertain about what they want to protect children from.

The key point, however, is that these tensions are not primarily to do with the needs of children, but with the moral conflicts of parents – conflicts that reflect the inherent contradictions of modern views of childhood. Parents worship children, but also seek to mould them; they value children's 'natural' spontaneity and self-expression, but only if it takes acceptable forms; they use commercial culture to build emotional connections with their children, but attack it (or feel guilty) when that bond breaks down. Meanwhile, Cross suggests, adults seek the cute and the cool not only in their children but also in themselves.

Yet as all these authors suggest, there is also an implicit class dimension to these concerns. The idealized images of 'wondrous innocence' are largely those of children from the wealthy middle and upper classes, while the 'rowdy' street culture of public amusements and popular media from which they need to be sheltered is primarily that of the urban working class. Likewise, the marketing appeals of advertisements for educational toys and well-equipped playrooms are essentially addressed to the suburban middle classes, or those who aspire to join them. Yet while middle-class parents might believe themselves to be escaping or resisting commercial culture – in the name of educational or cultural value, or indeed of natural childhood innocence – it is clear that these motivations too have been consistently commodified. As Ellen Seiter (1993) suggests, 'commercialism' is not just a property of cheap plastic toys, but also of the wooden ones favoured by the middle classes; it is not confined to Barbie and Bratz dolls, or to the TV merchandise that clogs the aisles of Toys 'R' Us, but applies equally to the nostalgic (and much more expensive) 'quality toys' that are available in upmarket stores; it is not only about mass-market operations like Mattel and Hasbro, but also about 'niche' educational toy companies such as Fisher Price and the Early Learning Centre.

The 'empowerment' of the child consumer

Cross's account of the changing strategies of the toy industry is echoed in Dan Cook's (2004) analysis of the children's clothing market. The mass production of clothes for children appeared somewhat later than that of toys and children's books, and did not fully emerge as a separate market in the United States until the 1910s. Drawing particularly on an analysis of trade publications, Cook traces a change in the first half of the twentieth century, in which marketers gradually shifted their attention away from parents (that is, mothers) towards children themselves. In the 1910s and 1920s, the mother was the key purchaser, and the buying of clothes was represented as an act of instinctive love and care. The marketing of clothing was infused with expert claims about children's welfare, and the clothing sections of department stores even provided advice and instruction in parenting. As with toy marketing, children's consumption was thereby somehow removed from the taint of commercial corruption. However, by the 1930s and 1940s, the approach had become much more child-centred. In seeking to take the child's point of view – and espousing what Cook calls 'pediocularity' – merchants, marketers and retailers came to regard children as consumers in their own right. Marketing publications and advertising appeals celebrated children's autonomy and agency: the child consumer was represented as 'willful, knowledgeable and desiring'. This change was also apparent in the design of products and packaging, shop displays and layouts, and the growth of market research on children. Children were still seen to need training in 'correct' consumer behaviour, which was characterized by modesty, restraint and simplicity; but they were also seen to have the right to exercise choice and to display their individuality.

As Lisa Jacobson (2004) suggests, this apparent 'empowerment' of the child consumer reflected emerging cultural ideals of children as active, independent and autonomous. Jacobson argues that the celebration of childhood innocence in early twentieth-century advertising was increasingly cut across by a more transgressive view of them as savvy and discerning consumers 'with bountiful and insistent consumer appetites'. By the 1920s, she suggests, this view had come to dominate: advertisers began to address children more directly, not least as a potential influence on their parents' consumer choices; and retailers were increasingly being urged to regard children as 'exacting' customers, who deserved to be treated with dignity rather than patronized.

As both Cook and Jacobson describe, the new emphasis on children's autonomy as consumers was also manifested in the use of more playful and 'participatory' approaches to marketing. Jacobson's most telling example is the American 'radio clubs' of the late 1920s and early 1930s, which sought to involve children in imaginative play and interaction with dramatic storylines, as well as quizzes and competitions. Part of the appeal was that the 'club' excluded adults: it addressed children directly, rather than their mothers, offering a child-only world rich in fantasy and mystery, whose secrets (for example in the form of special codes and shared intrigues) must be protected – not least from prying adults. As the costs of production rose, the programmes themselves were increasingly developed and produced by advertising agencies. Marketers also connected plot-lines to premium offers, which were only available through sending proofs of purchase; and this in turn led to increasing pressure on parents to buy specific products – causing many to resist what they perceived as exploitation and an attack on their buying authority. Ultimately, Jacobson suggests, children themselves were also disappointed, finding that the premium gifts rarely lived up to their promise. As this implies, there were distinct limits to the kinds of 'empowerment' that were on offer to children. However, it also suggests that some of the more 'participatory' techniques and strategies that are seen as characteristic of contemporary marketing – such as interactivity, child-centredness and the blurring of commercial and other content – are in fact far from new.

Segmenting the market: age and gender

A further key dimension here was the growing segmentation of the children's market. Dividing the market by age allowed marketers to target their sales pitches more accurately; but it also, of course, encouraged consumption, as products that were perceived (by children or by parents) as 'too young' could be cast off in favour of those that were defined as age-appropriate. As Cook (2004) suggests, the mid twentieth century saw marketers making increasingly fine-grained distinctions between different age categories – distinctions that were undoubtedly reinforced by the contemporary emergence of age-grading in schools, and by the popularization of 'age and stage' theories of child development. These new age-defined categories were manifested in products themselves, but also in

marketing appeals and in the physical organization
of children's clothing, age differences were not simply
about style and design; and the appropriateness of a garment
through its differentiation from those aimed at children who
older and younger – although children were also encouraged
forward, and to emulate the styles of their older peers.

Thus, Cook (2004) traces the emergence of the 'toddler' as a new
marketing category in the 1930s, a figure popularized in the media via child
stars such as Shirley Temple, and in the popular psychological theories of
parental advice literature. The unique physical and personality characteristics
of the toddler came to be defined through the wearing of a particular style
of clothing, especially for girls. Here again, Cook suggests, the child was
perceived as an active consumer, articulating specific wishes and desires,
and seeking products that would apparently express its individual
personality. In effect, the market invented a new phase in the life course,
while purporting merely to be responding to children's innate characteristics
and needs. Similar processes can be observed in more recent times – in the
invention of the 'teenager' as a marketing category in the late 1940s, the
'subteen' or 'pre-teen' in the 1950s, and more recently in the emergence
of the 'tween'.

Gender has been the other most obvious aspect of this segmenting of
the children's market: as any visit to a toy store will instantly show, this is
very much a 'pink and blue' world. While right-thinking parents frequently
bemoan the gendered polarization of the children's market, it is by no
means a new development – and indeed it is debatable whether it has
increased over time, as is often alleged. As Cross (1997) describes, the toy
market of the late nineteenth and early twentieth centuries was clearly
divided along gender lines: boys' toys focused on technology and war,
while girls were sold dolls – although he suggests that this was not
necessarily reflected in the actual preferences of children, which were
much less polarized.

Jacobson (2004) argues that the marketers and advertisers of the early
twentieth century tended to regard girls as more flexible, and boys as far
more rigid, in their gender identification – a position that certainly coincides
with the perceptions of some more contemporary marketers (e.g.
Schneider, 1987; Siegel et al., 2001). As such, there was more to be gained
from targeting boys, while girls did not need to be catered for so explicitly.
However, Jacobson also argues that the fundamental struggle for marketers
in the early part of the twentieth century was to revise the popular
conception of consumption as a feminine domain – and indeed as an

...of stores. In the case
...ent was defined
...bout size, but also
...were both
...to look

lebrating the (white, middle-class) boy
to align consumption with robust,
dvertising for mechanical toys as well as
ed boy consumer was represented as a
neur and consumer expert. According to
consumption also helped to shore up
rofessional legitimacy and their self-image
nity'. The heroic boy consumer was also
niddle-class egalitarian family: consumption
bond with their fathers, as well as an arena
:ise influence on their parents.

ggests, marketing to teenage girls typically
encouraged them   occupied with physical beauty as a means to
ensure popularity within the peer group. While active, athletic girls were
evident in some early twentieth-century advertising, during the 1930s they
began to give way to a view of feminine consumption as an essentially
domesticated, privatized domain. Adolescent girls were 'enmeshed in a
narcissistic world of self-surveillance' constructed not only by advertisers
but also by popular advice columnists, and played out in the complex social
hierarchies of the American high school. However, as Jacobson suggests,
in more recent years marketers have been much more inclined to see girls
as cultural trendsetters: it is no longer adequate to address boys and simply
expect that girls will follow (Jacobson, 2004: 221).

These accounts might be seen as evidence of the power of the market
to define and impose particular identities on children. Yet they can also be
seen to reflect an ongoing uncertainty on the part of marketers: there is a
recurring sense throughout this history of the children's market as
somehow inherently volatile and difficult to control. In certain sectors –
most notably toys – the rate of failure of new products has always been
comparatively high; and while enormous profits can undoubtedly be made,
these are in no way guaranteed. Segmenting the children's market into
specific 'niches' based on age or gender might thus be seen to represent an
attempt at risk management – although it too is fraught with difficulties,
not least because it correspondingly reduces the size of the potential
market. For example, recent attempts to launch specialist television
channels for boys and girls have so far failed; and, as we shall see in chapter
5, the phenomenon of 'age compression' (or 'kids getting older younger')
is one that marketers have found quite challenging to track and control.

As this implies, we should be wary of assuming that these attempts to
define consumer identities are necessarily successful. All the accounts I
have discussed here are largely based on evidence from producers –

companies, marketers, retailers and others. Yet real children are different from the children of marketers' imaginations, and they may well resist or refuse to recognize the categories that marketers construct. At least for younger children, parents are also likely to remain a powerful part of the equation here; and as we have seen, their definitions of desirable childhood identities may well conflict with those of the marketers. This is bound to result in a process of negotiation – both within the family and within the peer group – that can be fraught with difficulty; and the identity – or, more accurately, the plural identities – of the child consumer may often prove to be mutable and difficult to pin down. These issues are explored in more detail in chapters 7, 8 and 9.

Consumption across cultures

It should be noted that almost all the accounts considered here relate to the United States. There has been very little attempt to document the history of children's consumption outside this context, yet its extent and nature are likely to vary significantly in different national settings. Tora Korsvold's work on children's consumption in Norway makes an interesting contrast in this respect (Korsvold, 2010, in press). The history here is one of a strong welfare state, with significant limits on consumption: the image of the frugal, responsible consumer was particularly strong in the decades following the Second World War (when many 'luxury' commodities were still rationed), and has seen some resurgence more recently with the contemporary environmentalist movement. There is strong state-provided childcare for very young children, and a 'good childhood' is typically identified with nature and an active, outdoor life. At the same time, the discovery of oil and gas reserves has resulted in a precipitous rise in wealth: Norway is one of the most affluent countries in the world in terms of per capita income, yet it is also one of the most egalitarian.

In this context, both consumption and childhood have somewhat different meanings from those that are dominant in the United States – although Norway, of course, also participates in global markets. This has resulted in some interesting differences – and indeed dilemmas – in terms of consumption. The marketing of toys, for example, may reflect a greater emphasis on educational values (Korsvold, 2010), while the marketing of children's clothing focuses more on qualities of nature and physical fitness, for girls as well as boys (Korsvold, in press). Advertising for children's products also appears more inclined to stress functionality rather than qualities of design, even compared with that in other European countries (Husen, 2009). Meanwhile, the conspicuous consumption of the very wealthy is perceived with some disapproval in light of the dominant cultural emphasis on egalitarianism.

A very different comparison is possible with China, which has made the transition to a consumer society even more recently and rapidly. By comparison with Norway and with the United States, economic inequalities here are significantly more marked. Parents' views of children's consumption reflect some of the same anxieties and ambivalences felt by Western parents, but they are also inflected with very different values – for example about moderation and the difference between 'good' and 'bad' consumption – deriving from Confucianism (Waerdahl, 2010). On the other hand, the 'one child' policy may have led to some children enjoying considerable power as 'little emperors' of consumption within the family (McNeal and Yeh, 2003; Zhao and Murdock, 1996).

While not explicitly concerned with children, Ritty Lukose's (2009) ethnographic study of young people in the Indian state of Kerala points to some of the complexities that characterize such historical transformations. On one level, Lukose provides further evidence of the rise of Western-style 'consumerism' – in the form of fashion, movies, beauty pageants and ice cream parlours – in the global South; but she also refuses any simple view of this as a matter of 'Westernization' or 'modernization'. As she suggests, neo-liberalism has given rise to complex forms of cultural politics, in which consumption and citizenship have become intertwined, reconfiguring established relations of class (or caste) and gender, forms of public life and notions of national identity. As she shows, such developments offer new freedoms as well as new constraints, and they are by no means uncontested.

There are obviously very limited grounds for comparison here, and research from outside Western countries is still extremely scarce. However, the key point is that the status, extent and nature of children's consumption are likely to vary significantly, depending on wider cultural definitions both of consumption and of childhood. The United States' development as a consumer society certainly happened earlier than that of other countries, but it should not be taken to represent the norm.

A narrative of decline?

It would be easy to interpret the history of children's consumption as one of steady cultural decline. It could be argued that the 'commercialization' of childhood has undermined the power and authority of parents, and corrupted the natural innocence and purity of children themselves. Stephen

Kline's account, briefly discussed in chapter 3, exemplifies this approach: indeed, it is aptly summed up in the title of his book, *Out of the Garden* (1993). Kline's is to some extent a literal garden – a peaceful location where children apparently used to play freely until they were seduced indoors by the mesmerizing power of television. However, it is also a figurative one – a Garden of Eden, a space of purity and innocence that has been steadily invaded and destroyed by market forces. For Kline, the path from the 'simple delight' and 'artistic freedom' of nineteenth-century children's books to the 'mind-numbing banality' of contemporary TV cartoons is one that runs precipitously downhill.

There is perhaps a hint of this view in Gary Cross's account of the contemporary toy market – and especially in his more recent criticism of the role of consumer culture in infantilizing adult men (Cross, 2008). However, most of the historical accounts I have considered here suggest that the trajectory of historical change is rather more complex, and indeed more contradictory. Recent studies – such as those of Denisoff and his colleagues (2008) – suggest that the Golden Age whose loss Kline laments was far from free of commercial interests. As Cook (2004) argues, it is not that the market has somehow invaded or colonized childhood, or that childhood itself can be imagined as essentially non-commercial. Rather, the construction of childhood, and indeed of parenthood, is inextricable from the operations of the market.

Neither should this be conceived as a one-way process. On the contrary, it is characterized by ambivalence and uncertainty, and by an ongoing negotiation – even a struggle for power – between the imperatives of marketers, parents and children themselves. As Cross (1997) argues, the story is not simply one of marketers manipulating parents or exploiting children. Rather, we need to understand children's consumption in the context of broader social and cultural changes.

Thus, several of these studies suggest that changes in marketing to children reflected and reinforced parallel changes in family life, and in popular ideas about parenting. This is partly a consequence of demographic change – although here again, the picture is an ambivalent one. The steady decline in family size, and the general rise in disposable income, over the past century has meant that parents have more money to spend on their children, and yet that children may also have fewer playmates available to them in the home. On the other hand, the increasing involvement of women in the workplace means that parents may be less available to become involved in their children's play, or at least to stimulate it. Most children today have much greater spending power, and much more money spent on them, than their parents did when they were young – and this in itself can provoke complex feelings of displacement, resentment and guilt.

Meanwhile, as the studies by Seiter (1993) and Jacobson (2004) indicate, marketing to parents has increasingly been implicated with expert advice literature on child development – to the point where the two are sometimes hard to disentangle. Such literature typically proclaims a democratic, 'companionate' approach to child rearing; but it also places a central responsibility on parents (or specifically mothers) for ensuring their child's healthy development and eventual success in life. This particular combination of advice seems almost designed to provoke greater consumption, perhaps particularly among middle-class parents. Buying stuff for your children can be a convenient way of appearing to meet their needs; it can help to avoid disputes, and reward obedience; it can address educational objectives, provided one believes the marketing claims about the pedagogic value of the products; and it can assuage one's own guilt in being unable to provide sufficient 'quality time'.

Yet the greatest paradox here is that children's new status as consumers is indicative of a broader and more fundamental shift in social power. The rise of the child consumer coincides with, and feeds upon, the growing enfranchisement of the child – and, as we have seen, the notion of the child as active and empowered is one that has frequently been espoused by marketers (Cook, 2004). Over the past century, we have steadily come to regard children not as vulnerable innocents, but as social actors in their own right. The child's point of view is not to be ignored, but respected and taken into account: children are seen to have the right to make choices, to express their views and desires, and to have their voices heard. Yet this has been an uneven development, which has provoked considerable anxiety on the part of adults. And one of the primary reasons for this anxiety is because it has been driven, not only by social welfare campaigners or progressive forces in society, but also – and some would say predominantly – by the market.

As we shall see in the following chapter, marketing to children has changed significantly in recent times. Children are being targeted in many new ways, and they have vastly increased opportunities to consume. The abiding question, however, is about the nature and extent of the 'empowerment' this might afford. Children are by no means all equal here. Indeed, it could well be argued that markets tend to accentuate inequalities, or at least the subjective experience of inequality. As a social group, children may in general have become more powerful – but what are the consequences if that growing power is ultimately just the power to consume?

5

The contemporary ch

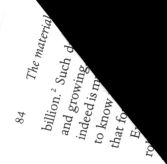

While there is a long history of marketing to c... remarkable step change in the past two decades. The size or ... market appears to have grown significantly. The range of commerci... products and services available to them has massively expanded, and they are being targeted as consumers at an ever-younger age. Marketing now increasingly addresses children directly: it occurs through a much wider range of media, and in a wider range of settings, some of which have hitherto been largely insulated from the operations of the market.

However, this image of a growing market is not easy to quantify. For different reasons, both marketers and campaigners seem inclined to 'talk up' the size of the children's market, resulting in figures that are sometimes quite astronomical. Lindstrom and Seybold (2003), for example, estimate that US children aged 8–14 spend around $150 billion annually, 'control' another $150 billion of their parents' money, and influence family spending of up to $600 billion a year. Meanwhile, they suggest, the global children's market is worth something approaching $2 *trillion*. It is difficult to obtain reliable or meaningful information in this area, perhaps partly because of commercial confidentiality, but also because some industries do not gather or segment data relating specifically to children. One indicative figure here is that of the total cost of bringing up a child, which is measured annually in the UK by a leading insurance company: in 2010 this figure topped £200,000, representing an increase of over 40 per cent across the last five years.[1] On this basis, the cost of bringing up all children in the UK born in 2007 would be £134 billion (not including inflation).

Figures on children's discretionary spending are quite variable, although one fairly cautious set of estimates suggests that British children under the age of 16 spend £680 million of their own money on snacks and sweets every year, followed by clothing (£660 m), music and CDs (£620 m), footwear (£400 m), computer software and games (£350 m), magazines (£250 m) and toiletries (£83 m). These figures need to be set in the context of total UK consumer expenditure, which in 2007 amounted to £875

azzling numbers clearly confirm that the market is large
although it is hard to know whether it is growing faster (or
uch more profitable) than other market sectors. It is also difficult
whether particular sub-sectors of the children's market – such as
pre-school children – are in fact expanding relative to others.

xperts on children's marketing typically see them as playing three
les here (McNeal, 1992, 1999). Most obviously, they are consumers in
their own right, spending their disposable income on their own behalf
(albeit with the influence of peers and parents). Secondly, they also act as
influences on family purchasing; and while this is sometimes presented as
a matter of 'pester power', it is not always a matter of direct appeals, nor
indeed is it necessarily about 'pestering' (as we shall see in chapter 8).
Finally, children are seen to represent long-term 'market potential':
marketers may seek to cultivate brand loyalty, in the expectation that this
will pay off in the future. These roles are reflected in the whole range of
marketing and promotional appeals that target children. They are apparent
not only in the advertisements for toys or breakfast cereals on children's
television, but also in the many ads for cars or financial services that feature
children – and indeed in the intensive marketing of educational goods and
services to parents.

As we have seen, the long-term growth of the children's market needs
to be understood in the context of broader changes in family life, and in
society more broadly. Particularly over the past fifty years, industrialized
societies have experienced rising affluence and prosperity – although this
has been very unevenly distributed. The size of families has dropped, and
parents are having children later in life. There has been a rise in single-
parent families, and in families where both parents are working; and greater
longevity means that more children have living grandparents. All these
developments are likely to result in children becoming more prominent,
both as consumers in their own right and as influences on family decision-
making. This has in turn been reinforced by changing ideas about child
rearing, which have tended to stress the need for parents to protect and
invest in their children, while simultaneously calling for a more equal
balance of power within the family. These issues will be discussed in more
detail in chapter 8.

Empowered consumers?

One index of the growth of this market has been the explosion of marketing
discourse specifically concerned with children. Again, this is not a new
development (Cook, 2000; Kline, 1993), but it is one that has vastly increased

in scope and scale over the past decade. There has been a proliferation of new companies concerned with tracking and targeting the children's market; many advertising, marketing and PR companies now have divisions or units specializing in this field; significantly more is being spent on market research with children; and there is a growing world of industry conferences and award shows specifically concerned with children's marketing (see Schor, 2004).

As we saw in chapter 1, contemporary marketers have been keen to present the growth of the children's market as a matter of the 'empowerment' of children. The work of historians such as Jacobson (2004) and Cook (2004) shows that this is in fact a longer-term development: the modern image of the active, desiring and autonomous child consumer has its roots in the new marketing discourses that rose to prominence in the 1920s and 1930s (at least in the United States). Yet contemporary marketers make even greater play of children's power and knowledge as consumers (e.g. del Vecchio, 1997; Lindstrom and Seybold, 2003; Sutherland and Thompson, 2001). Kids today, they tell us, are savvy and sophisticated; they can recognize when advertisers are trying to manipulate them; they are quick to adopt new trends, but also quick to move on; they expect to be treated with respect, and not patronized; they know what they like, what they want, and how to get it.

According to Canadian marketers Anne Sutherland and Beth Thompson (2001: 3), children today 'control more of their destiny than possibly at any other time in history': 'Kids today want to be heard and they will make sure that corporations listen. Kids today are empowered, and they are experiencing the world from the bottom up, rather than the top down ... Kids are knocking on the world's door, saying speak *with* me – not at me' (p. 178).

As I have noted, such arguments implicitly align the growing status of children as consumers with broader arguments about children's rights. According to these authors, children's new-found power is not just about buying and selling, but also about 'kids wanting to have a say about things that affect their lives, present and future' (p. 117). Yet the power children are seen to enjoy here derives primarily from the power to spend money: Sutherland and Thompson's notion of 'kidfluence' refers not only to *influence* but also to *affluence*. In some instances, this celebration of children's power also slides across into an explicit resistance towards, or rejection of, adults' perspectives: 'anti-adultism' appears to be a persuasive rhetoric both in the statements of marketers and in the kinds of appeals that are addressed to children themselves (see Banet-Weiser, 2007; Kinder, 1991; Seiter, 1993).

Contemporary marketing texts often seek to explain the development of the children's market in terms of a popular historical narrative of generational change in the United States (the 'boomers' are followed by 'the baby bust', by Generations X and Y, and so on). Children are routinely seen here as a 'digital generation', with an apparently spontaneous expertise in their dealings with technology. They no longer seem to be regarded as gullible, or as a 'soft touch' – not least because of their increasing exposure to marketing itself. Children, we are told, are also subject to the phenomenon of 'age compression': they are 'getting older younger' – partly because of an adult-driven pressure to compete, but also because of their growing access to aspects of adult life that were formerly hidden from view. This appears to be particularly the case for the newly identified category of the 'tween' – described by Siegel et al. (2001: 4) as having 'a "split personality" which toggles between kid behaviors and attitudes and those of a teenager'.

Yet for all this emphasis on change, marketers are also advised to address needs that are seen as somehow timeless – needs for mastery, stability, fantasy, romance and rebellion (and so on). Many of these marketing texts rely on mechanistic 'age and stage' models of child development – Piaget is alive and well here too – and on notions of innate human need derived from Maslow's 'hierarchy of needs' (see chapter 2). These innate needs remain quite strikingly gendered, and in some instances they vary between different types of child consumers. Lindstrom and Seybold (2003), for example, differentiate between persuaders, followers, 'edges' and reflexives, each of which is seen to have different tastes and purchasing habits. Children at different ages are seen to be 'looking for an identity', seeking 'to identify with a role model' or beginning 'to develop and understand their personal power in the world' – and marketers must seek to understand such needs in order to identify when children are most 'brand aware' and 'open to suggestion' (Sutherland and Thompson, 2001). Siegel et al. (2001) invoke both Piaget and Maslow in asserting that tweens seek 'power, freedom, fun and belonging', are very oriented towards detail, and have a strong desire to learn – and they seek to exemplify the ways in which particular marketing campaigns have addressed these characteristics. Yet for all their scientific legitimation, it is hard to imagine that such generalized proposals might prove especially useful.

Critics of marketing to children tend to dismiss this emphasis on empowerment as a form of superficial public relations (e.g. Schor, 2004). As they suggest, such arguments are routinely used by marketers to displace public criticism – along with the recurrent assertion that the responsibility for regulating children's consumption is a matter for parents, rather than for the market itself (or indeed for government). Yet in the marketing texts, the assertion of empowerment also sits rather awkwardly alongside a continuing emphasis on children's emotional and psychological fears and vulnerabilities at different ages – and advice to marketers on how they might usefully tap into them. Among tweens, for example, a key source of anxiety is seen to relate to their social status among the peer group: marketing appeals that promise to help them 'fit in' are thus regarded as especially powerful at this age. These books overflow with suggestions on how to target and manipulate children, both through marketing appeals and through new 'kid-oriented' products – and indeed on how to exploit parents' concerns as well. Children are seen as powerful, but they are also often described in almost Pavlovian terms, as displaying programmed responses to particular marketing appeals or sensory signals, and in constant pursuit of instant gratification.

Media and cultural industries: the bigger picture

While the growth of the children's market does need to be understood in the context of changes in family life, it also needs to be related to broader developments in the media and cultural industries. Media are, of course, commodities in themselves: as the figures above suggest, a very significant part of the children's market relates to media, either in the form of physical objects that are owned (computer games, CDs, magazines, books) or in the form of experiences (visits to the cinema, subscriptions to cable TV or internet services, trips to theme parks). This market is undoubtedly proliferating, as can be seen from the massive expansion in the number of specialist children's television channels that have appeared in the past fifteen years (there are currently around thirty in the UK). Meanwhile, the commercial success of most other children's products – such as toys, clothing or food – is increasingly dependent upon media exposure, although this goes a long way beyond advertising per se. Children's consumption, we might say, is almost invariably *mediated* consumption.

A detailed discussion of broader developments in these areas is beyond the scope of this book, but a number of general tendencies can be briefly identified here (comprehensive recent accounts may be found, for example, in Hesmondhalgh (2007) and Lash and Lury (2007)). Perhaps the most immediately obvious changes here have been to do with technology. Over the past twenty years, digitization has led to the emergence of a whole range of new technologies of production, distribution and consumption. Previously distinct media forms and commodities have begun to converge, as television programmes are linked to websites, films and computer games – and, of course, to merchandising and advertising. Indeed, it is possible to argue that many media texts have effectively become advertisements for other texts: seeing the film encourages us to buy the game or the merchandise, and vice versa. Companies are increasingly operating across media platforms and markets, rather than specializing in particular areas; and success is more and more dependent upon visibility in a range of media.

Meanwhile, access to media has become increasingly individualized. For example, the majority of children in the UK now have televisions, DVD players, games consoles and computers (increasingly with internet access) in their bedrooms, as well as portable media devices such as mobile phones and iPods. As media, products and services have proliferated, markets have begun to fragment. As a result, marketers are increasingly bound to address 'niche' audiences – and to attempt to amass such audiences on a global scale. As consumers' tastes have become more diverse and less predictable, targeting audiences has become a more complex and difficult process, and this has led to a growing emphasis both on marketing itself and on various forms of market research and data-gathering (Arvidsson, 2006).

Markets have also become increasingly globalized, and while there has been a concentration of ownership into large transnational companies, there has also been a rise in the number of smaller companies, and in casual or freelance labour. Broadly speaking, the proliferation of media and of goods and services has meant that markets are now increasingly competitive: while great profits can undoubtedly be made from successful properties – particularly if these are played out across a range of media platforms and markets – the likelihood of commercial failure in many sectors is very high. The imperative for companies has now become one of managing risk – for example, through capitalizing on past or existing successes, and through various kinds of formatting and branding.

Nearly all these media are commercially provided and funded. Public service media have generally declined, or been compelled to adopt more commercially oriented approaches, while the state regulation of media has become less and less significant. In many instances, the boundaries between promotional material and 'editorial' or other content have become increasingly blurred; and while this is most overtly the case with product placement, commercial considerations are also increasingly important in determining themes, narratives and forms of representation across a wide range of media genres. Advertising and marketing have become ubiquitous, both in electronic and print media and in public spaces – although, as we shall see below, marketers are now more likely to use less direct or visible approaches (such as sponsorship and peer-to-peer marketing) rather than traditional 'hard sell' tactics. Consumers are increasingly addressed as active agents, rather than as malleable or as easily duped; and new techniques, for example based on 'viral', 'personalized' or 'participatory' marketing, have become increasingly significant as means of leveraging that agency and putting it to work. Branding has also become a particularly important strategy here: 'brand equity' can be transferred across and between different markets, and consumers themselves become active participants in producing and disseminating the meanings of brands – albeit in ways that companies must constantly seek to manage (Arvidsson, 2006; Lury, 2004)

From tie-ins to programme-length commercials to integrated marketing

The complex web of economic, technological and cultural factors that I have very briefly sketched here is perhaps most apparent in the success of the children's media 'crazes' of the 1990s and 2000s, like *Teenage Mutant Ninja Turtles*, Pokémon, Harry Potter or *High School Musical* (see Kinder, 1991; Tobin, 2004). In fact, such cross-media marketing – sometimes referred to as 'integrated marketing' – is far from being a recent development. Disney is of course the best-known example of this phenomenon: right from the early days of the Mickey Mouse clubs (which began in cinemas in the 1930s, and came to television in the mid-1950s), merchandising has been an indispensable aspect of the enterprise, and has even sometimes served to keep the media production operation afloat (see Bryman, 1995; de Cordova, 1994; Wasko, 2001). Such strategies were also apparent in the early days of British public broadcasting, where the figures of Muffin the Mule and Sooty (both notably revived in recent years) became lucrative vehicles for spin-off merchandising. Smith (2010) discusses a much earlier instance of cross-media marketing in the form of the 'Bubble books', story books with recordings attached, which were produced by RCA Victor in the early 1900s; while, in the mid eighteenth century, one of the pioneers of children's publishing, John Newbery, regularly sold his books with 'free gifts' – such as pin-cushions, balls and even headache tonics – to boost sales (Thomas, 2007: 163).

Even so, the late 1970s is often taken to be an important watershed in the emergence of media-related merchandising (see Clark, 2007; Cross, 1997; Engelhardt, 1986; Kline, 1993). It was at this point that toy companies in particular became much more centrally involved in the production of media for children. The first attempts in this direction were made in the late 1960s, when the toy company Hasbro created an animated TV series based on its Hot Wheels range. The programme was disallowed by the US Federal Communications Commission (FCC), on the grounds that it would 'subordinate programming in the interests of the public to programming in the interests of its saleability'. However, with the subsequent deregulation of television under the Reagan administration, the FCC adopted a much more 'free market' stance (Kunkel, 1988), and so began the era of what critics came to call 'programme-length commercials'. Leading toy companies such as Mattel and Hasbro commissioned animated series – such as *Thundercats*, *Transformers*, *Care Bears* and *Smurfs* – that were sold cheaply to the networks, and effectively served as shop-windows for their extensive ranges of collectable toys and accessories. In some cases, toy companies even offered TV stations royalties on sales in exchange for time slots (Cross, 1997: 201).

As Cross (1997) suggests, such programmes offered toy manufacturers the possibility of managing a toy 'craze', for example by gradually exposing new additions to the range. This kind of co-ordinated approach was particularly crucial given the apparent volatility of the children's market, and relatively low profit margins. For critics, however, programme-length commercials effectively 'scripted' children's play, confining them to a mere imitation of pre-defined scenarios, and effectively undermining free, imaginative play (Kline, 1993) – although such arguments were only partly borne out by research (e.g. Greenfield et al., 1990).

The concept of media tie-ins was not confined to television: indeed, it also owed a lot to another contemporary success, George Lucas's *Star Wars* (1977). However, the differences with the programme-length commercials were that in the latter the products were created *before* the media texts, rather than vice versa, and the toy companies were effectively the producers rather than subsequently being licensed to produce 'spin-offs'. In the intervening years, however, this distinction has become somewhat moot. In the case of Ninja Turtles and Harry Potter, it is possible to trace an 'original' text, existing independently of later media versions and merchandising tie-ins: indeed, in both cases, the success of that text (an underground comic and a book, respectively) appears to have taken their publishers or producers by surprise. However, in the case of Pokémon – which will be considered in more detail shortly – and subsequent multimedia 'crazes' such as Digimon, YuGiOh or Beyblades, this kind of integrated marketing appears to have been part of the plan from the outset. The presence of such branded merchandise in so many media and market sectors – including not just toys, but also clothing, food, gifts and other paraphernalia – effectively makes them impossible to avoid, generating a 'virtuous circle' of ubiquitous mutual promotion. This approach has now effectively replaced 'programme-length commercials' in their original form; and it is now by no means confined to animation, as the continuing success of franchises such as Harry Potter, Disney's *High School Musical* and *Hannah Montana*, and the BBC's *Doctor Who* clearly illustrates.

Indeed, integrated marketing has been crucial to many of the most popular children's television series of the past ten years or so. Character licensing – from Bob the Builder and Thomas the Tank Engine to Dora the Explorer and Tickle Me Elmo – is an increasingly crucial strategy in terms of managing the children's market: characters are effectively the children's equivalent of brands, and they can be deployed and circulated across a wide range of products, from media and toys to food and clothing. Meanwhile, a programme like *Teletubbies*, which required a very large initial investment, would almost certainly not have been produced without the company (in this case, the independent Ragdoll, working for the BBC) being able to predict substantial revenue from merchandising and overseas programme sales (Buckingham, 2002a). Indeed, as this latter example illustrates, such considerations are by no means confined to the commercial sector. The extensive merchandising revenue generated from the American PBS show *Sesame Street* might also be cited as further evidence of the blurring of boundaries between public and commercial providers in the children's market – and, indeed, public service programming increasingly has to depend upon such revenue in order to survive. The implications of some of these developments in terms of broadcasting and other media will be considered in more detail in chapter 10.

Integrated marketing of this kind is by no means confined to the children's market, and, although it can offer considerable financial rewards, it remains a relatively high-risk strategy. Indeed, it is here that some of the volatility and unpredictability of the children's market becomes most apparent. The success of such phenomena often appears to take their producers by surprise, leading to shortages of the most sought-after products and queues of frustrated would-be buyers in the shops. Licensees, manufacturers and retailers will then frequently wade into the market, only to be left stranded – and often bankrupt – when the tide recedes.

The case of Pokémon

The example of Pokémon, the multimedia 'craze' that appeared to colonize the imaginations of a whole generation of children for a brief period around the turn of the millennium, illustrates many of these broader developments – as well as providing a further instance of the cultural studies approach introduced in chapter 3 (for more detail, see Buckingham and Sefton-Green, 2003; Tobin, 2004). At its peak in 2000, Pokémon was undoubtedly the most profitable children's 'craze' of all time: in that year, it reputedly generated over $7 billion worldwide. Beginning as a computer game, quickly followed by a TV series, a trading card game, feature films, books, magazines, toys and a plethora of other merchandise, Pokémon is the paradigm example of contemporary 'integrated marketing'. Yet two or three years later, it seemed to have been abruptly dropped: while new Pokémon products are still being produced, they no longer have anything like the ubiquity or the central position in children's culture they once enjoyed – although the manufacturers have frequently attempted to recycle them for subsequent generations.

There are different ways of accounting for the success of Pokémon. To some extent, it can be seen as a very calculated commercial strategy on the part of its originators, the Nintendo Corporation of Japan. In targeting the game at the children's market, rather than the youth market dominated by Sony, and in devising a product that would effectively exploit the unique qualities of its Game Boy hand-held console, Nintendo was playing to its strengths. Taken as a whole, Pokémon products seem to have been designed to maximize appeal across the traditionally fragmented children's market. The products combined conventional 'girl appeal' (via an emphasis on nurturing and 'cuteness') with 'boy appeal' (via the emphasis on collecting and competition). Different types of products were also targeted at different age groups – soft toys for younger children, TV cartoons for 6- to 8-year-olds, computer games for older children – allowing children to 'graduate' from one to the next.

On the other hand, Pokémon is often described as the product of an individual 'creator', Satoshi Tajiri; and in designing the game, Tajiri apparently set out to recapture elements of his own childhood (such as his fascination with collecting insects). According to this account, the success of Pokémon was somewhat unpredictable: it 'took off' because children somehow instinctively recognized and responded to Tajiri's personal vision. There is obviously an element of mythology about this account. Nevertheless, as with previous 'crazes' of this kind, the companies involved were somewhat slow to respond to this immediate popularity; and the eventual demise of Pokémon – which was even more precipitous than its rise – was far from accurately predicted. These familiar patterns of rise and fall in children's 'crazes' are difficult to explain if we regard them simply as a matter of corporate manipulation.

The central narrative of Pokémon is that of the hero's quest. The 10-year-old Ash leaves home in search of the mythical creatures that will eventually bring him adult mastery. Assisted by various helpers and donors, he travels uncharted lands encountering a series of obstacles and enemies, until (at least in the computer games) he finally arrives at his goal and defeats his rival trainers. In doing so, he must learn to overcome his emotional side, and achieve self-control. In this respect, the appeal of Pokémon is similar to that of many other stories of masculine maturation, which recur not just in classic children's literature but also in martial arts movies, role-playing games and fantasy novels. In some respects, Pokémon could be seen as a form of training in the characteristic cultural forms of male adolescence – although, as I have noted, it also has things in common with 'girl culture', such as the 'maternal' appeal of collectable toys and Tamagotchis.

Knowledge – or at least the acquisition of information – is central to the whole phenomenon. Significantly, much of this knowledge is inaccessible and meaningless to non-initiates – most obviously, adults. This knowledge is also designed to be portable across different media or platforms: what you learn from the TV cartoon can be usefully applied in the card game, and vice versa. This 'portability' allows different aspects of the phenomenon to be enjoyed in different social contexts, either alone or with others: it provides a useful way of 'filling in time' when no alternative options are available, and a 'ticket of entry' to play and friendship groups. More broadly, it can be argued that becoming part of the Pokémon culture involved actively seeking out new information and new products from a range of sources. Pokémon was not something you would merely 'read' or 'consume', but something you needed to *do* and to participate in.

Our research into the uses of Pokémon (Tobin, 2004) illustrates the diverse – and in some instances, highly creative – ways in which children consumed, appropriated and re-worked these products in different cultural settings. They actively interpreted the texts, relating them both to broader moral and social concerns (such as good and evil, or friendship and competition) and to specific local or national issues. In Israel, for example, the children picked up on the theme of 'fighting for peace', reflecting a national context characterized by ongoing military conflict (Lemish and Bloch, 2004); in Australia, Aboriginal children bypassed the competitive elements of the card game, and chose to play collaboratively; while in France, the children adapted the game for playing traditional French card games such as La Bataille and La Tapette (Brougère, 2004). Children also used the products and their knowledge of the Pokémon universe to create play scenarios of their own invention, in which Pokémon featured alongside other (seemingly randomly assembled) toys and artefacts; and in some instances, as in the UK, they created their own Pokémon-related texts (Bromley, 2004; Willett, 2004). Far from being passive consumers, children were using these texts selectively in their play, and re-inventing them for their own purposes.

On the other hand, there were certainly elements here that might be seen to involve the commercial exploitation of children. Children (including my own) were encouraged to spend large amounts of money in their efforts to collect rare trading cards – although this 'rarity' or scarcity was of course artificially created by the trading card companies. Some saw this process as a means of enabling children to learn valuable lessons about economic life – although, for others, it was tantamount to extortion (Cooper, 2000).

Even so, a phenomenon like Pokémon cannot be seen simply as a case of powerful corporations manipulating vulnerable children. Children do have some power to determine how the phenomenon evolves, the purposes it will serve, and the ways in which it can be used; and indeed – as they did in this case – they may drop it very quickly once it has outlived its interest and value for them. As I suggested in chapter 2, this should not be seen as an either/or choice, although *activity* on the part of audiences should not necessarily be equated with *agency* or power. Contemporary media phenomena like Pokémon position children as active participants, even if that activity is mediated almost entirely through commercial processes and relationships – and, as such, they may at least *feel* 'empowering', even if ultimately they are not.

In many of these respects, the case of Pokémon also exemplifies the globalization (or, more accurately, the 'glocalization') of children's markets. On the one hand, the products were consciously designed for global consumption, both at the point of production in Japan and at the point of distribution, as they were franchised out and adapted by other companies around the world. While some elements appeared distinctively Japanese, the visual style was a combination of Japanese and 'Western' conventions; and aspects that were perceived as 'too' Japanese – and hence as culturally strange – were mostly removed. Yet on the other hand, the products were also 'localized' by children themselves, in the ways in which they were appropriated in their play and in their everyday peer-group culture. In our research, we observed several instances of children communicating and playing with Pokémon across social and cultural differences: its extensive, specialized mythology provided a kind of common language that transcended cultural barriers. In this context, the 'Japaneseness' of Pokémon was something that children recognized and enjoyed: it was strange, but strange-exotic – and, indeed, profoundly cool (see McGray, 2002). Similar processes of 'glocalization' in children's consumer culture are apparent in the case of Disney products and of the Harry Potter phenomenon (for further discussion, see de Block and Buckingham, 2007).

Children's play ... and children's work

While these developments are perhaps most apparent in relation to children's media, they also apply to other areas of the children's market, such as toys. Eric Clark's journalistic exposé of the contemporary toy industry illustrates many of the broader tendencies identified earlier in this chapter (Clark, 2007). Clark estimates that the global toy industry is currently worth $69 billion annually, although this is an increasingly competitive business, serving a rapidly changing market – and to some extent, as children continue to 'get older younger', it is also a shrinking one. The proportion of new products that fail to generate profit is much higher than in many other sectors, and a great many ideas that are projected never make it beyond the initial development stage. The turn-around time for successful product lines has reduced, sales are still seasonally uneven, and profit margins are comparatively low.

In this uncertain context, companies have become increasingly dominated by what Clark calls a 'hit mentality'. Even so, losers massively outnumber winners, and risk management has effectively become the key imperative. Integrated marketing, strong branding and the incessant recycling of past successes (particularly those that capitalize on parents' nostalgia for the toys of their own childhood) have become crucial in the attempt to manage the market. The toy market has also become increasingly tied in with media markets: the large majority of the most popular toys are licensed or franchised products rather than generic ones. Since initial development and production costs for new toys are relatively high, it also makes much more sense to extend existing product ranges, and to rely on media tie-ins. Attempts to broaden brands or company profiles are fraught with difficulty, as the problems faced by the Lego company in its efforts to enter the 'mediatized' end of the global toy market over the past decade have suggested (Hjarvard, 2004). All this inevitably results in a reduction in the scope for innovation.

While the toy industry has historically included a significant proportion of independent, smaller-scale manufacturers and retailers, it is now increasingly dominated by a small number of very large global companies. The market leaders Mattel and Hasbro have swallowed up many smaller firms, while retailing is increasingly dominated by a few very large companies, most notably (in the United States and beyond) Wal-Mart and Toys 'R' Us, who are well known for their cut-throat discounting strategies. Such companies are also better placed than smaller firms to benefit from the media tie-ins that have become increasingly critical to success. Indeed, Clark (2007) estimates that as many as one-third of all toys in the United States are purchased in fast-food 'happy meals', most of which are in turn related to current media launches. Meanwhile, production is increasingly outsourced to Asia, and to sweatshop factories that are notorious for employment practices which are little better than slavery (Clark, 2007: ch. 8).

The battle between Barbie and the Bratz dolls illustrates many of the tensions that result from this increasingly precarious situation (Clark, 2007: ch. 4). Like Lego, Barbie is a long-established 'classic' toy whose supremacy as a market leader has become somewhat uncertain in recent times. While Barbie has undergone several transformations and adopted countless new careers over the years, the brand has remained remarkably consistent. Mattel, the producer, is ferociously protective of the brand – and indeed notoriously litigious towards those who have taken Barbie's name in vain. However, Barbie has failed to see off the challenge of the Bratz dolls, new entrants to the contemporary market who have ironically been condemned for many of the same reasons (to do with 'sexualization' in particular) that were originally applied to Barbie. In this context, Barbie runs the risk of appearing unattractively wholesome and old-fashioned, and significantly less than cool (cf. Cross, 2004). Meanwhile, the phenomenon of 'kids getting older younger' (KGOY in marketing-speak) means that the market for dolls is effectively being squeezed. Mattel's somewhat desperate attempts to reinvent Barbie, and to generate new product lines that will rival Bratz and reach out to new markets, have largely met with failure, at least thus far. (Elizabeth Chin's (2001) analysis of the company's misguided attempts to produce 'ethnically correct' dolls provides further evidence on this point.)

However, it would be wrong to assume that these pressures apply only to mass-market products, or to those that are deemed to be primarily about play. In another journalistic account, Susan Gregory Thomas (2007) provides an illuminating analysis of the growing market for young children's 'educational' toys and media, which displays many of the same characteristics. One market leader here is *Baby Einstein*, a range of 'developmental' DVDs aimed at under-2s, which has now generated a series of sub-brands in the form of *Baby Shakespeare, Baby Newton, Baby Mozart* and (implausibly enough) *Baby Van Gogh*. The company was founded in the late 1990s by an individual mother, but was bought five years later for an estimated $25 million by Disney. More recent entrants to this market include *Brainy Baby, Brilliant Baby* and *Smart Baby*, while a practical guide to using such approaches is symptomatically entitled *Baby Power: Give Your Child Real Learning Power* (Wade and Moore, 2000). Other examples would include the LeapPad, a dedicated computer console with a suite of associated 'learning system' software, as well as the extensive ranges of educational toys and products associated with television shows such as *Teletubbies, Blue's Clues* and *Dora the Explorer*, and with films such as Disney's Pooh series.

Of course, the primary market for these products is parents, rather than children. As Thomas (2007) describes, much of the marketing here depends on educational claims, which are often bolstered by the testimony of developmental psychologists and childcare experts. The marketing typically emphasizes 'creativity', 'discovery' and 'fun', and seeks to distance itself from the negative associations of 'hothousing' – and Thomas argues that this approach is particularly critical for 'Generation X' parents, who are likely to resist the 'hard sell'. Even so, the pedagogic intent of these products is quite narrowly defined: they are about 'fun', but they are also very definitely about learning – and indeed about learning conceived in fairly traditional terms, as a matter of the mastery of skills and the recall of facts. The role of infant neuroscience (or 'brain science') is especially crucial here: parents are repeatedly informed that the very young child's brain is at a critical stage in development, and that if neural pathways are not formed now, they will be closed forever (see also Nadesan, 2002). Ideas of this kind are also popularized in notions such as the 'Mozart effect', whereby playing classical music to young children (and, indeed, even to babies in the womb) is deemed to accelerate their development. However spurious or overstated such claims may be, it is certainly the case that the educational benefits of such products are very far from proven: at most, like other educational media, it would seem that any such benefit is only likely to be realized in the context of intensive mediation and involvement by parents.

Yet for children, as Thomas (2007) suggests, the key issue here is not to do with learning, but with branding and character licensing. The presence of licensed characters enables children to form 'personalized' connections with the products; and these are reinforced as children encounter the same characters, not only in learning software and TV shows, but also in their nursery schools and on trips to supermarkets and fast-food restaurants. As such, Thomas argues, the most significant kind of learning that is taking place here is actually to do with character recognition: it is about selling much more than about education.

Of course, the marketing of educational goods to parents is by no means new, nor indeed are the claims that are typically made about them (Cross, 1997; Jacobson, 2004). Similar academic analyses have also recently been undertaken in relation to 'educational' products for older children, such as books, magazines and computer software (see Buckingham and Scanlon, 2003, 2005; Ito, 2009; Seiter, 1993). On one level, the growth of this market could be seen as merely a further instance of capitalism's restless search for new markets – or indeed as another manifestation of the phenomenon of 'age compression'. However, it should also be seen as a symptom of the growing emphasis on competitiveness in education – particularly, but by no means exclusively, among middle-class parents (Buckingham and Scanlon, 2003; Vincent and Ball, 2007). In this new climate, parents are under increasing pressure to ensure that their children not only reach the required developmental milestones, but also *exceed* them – and thence gain entry to a 'good' school or a 'good' university. Yet this growing demand for parental involvement in education has arisen at a time when mothers are increasingly working outside the home, and when the form of family life is changing (via the rise in divorce and single parenthood). Particularly for parents who lead pressured lives, one solution is to throw money at the problem: paying for educational goods and services offers the promise of educational advantage which they may feel unable to secure on their own behalf, or in their own time. (These issues will be discussed in more detail in chapters 8 and 11.)

New tactics, new issues

In recent years, marketers have begun to develop a range of new techniques for addressing the growing unpredictability of the children's market. To some extent, these reflect broader tendencies in the cultural industries of the kind outlined earlier in this chapter, and many (though by no means all) of them are specifically related to the development of digital technology. In addition to the forms of integrated marketing described above, it is possible to identify a range of other promotional strategies, which would include:

- product placement: not in itself a new strategy, but nevertheless a practice that is becoming more widespread in a range of media, and has recently been legalized in UK television (albeit not in children's programmes);
- other methods of embedding commercial messages, for example through the use of advertising hoardings in computer sports games or online social worlds;
- viral marketing, whereby commercial messages (in the form of e-mails or SMS texts or images) are forwarded from one user to another;
- advergaming, whereby players are involved in games (most obviously on company websites) using commercial or branded imagery or content;
- 'immersive' marketing and the gathering of personal data in online social worlds, both subscription sites and 'free' branded ones;
- social networking – in particular, the use of 'applications' that involve users in competitions featuring branded products and services, the use of branded materials (such as 'skins' or backgrounds), and the ways in which users are invited to define and construct their personal profiles in terms of preferences for consumer goods;
- sponsorship: again, a well-established strategy but one that appears to be becoming more widespread, not least in the context of public institutions, events and services (see chapter 11);
- data mining: that is, the gathering and analysis of data about consumers based on their responses to online requests, or (more covertly) through the use of 'cookies' that track their movements online;
- peer-to-peer marketing, whereby opinion leaders are recruited and paid as 'brand champions' or 'ambassadors' who will actively display and advocate the use of particular products within their contact group (the ubiquitous display of logos on branded clothing might be seen as a 'softer' form of this practice);
- new forms of market research that involve visiting and studying children in their homes, or recruiting them to inform marketers about current trends within their peer group ('cool hunting');
- the commercial cultivation of forms of 'fan culture' that involve collecting commodities (often those with a market-induced 'rarity' value), or creating forms of fan 'art' (for example, creating and circulating re-edited video material);
- so-called 'user-generated content', in which companies recruit consumers to create blogs or online videos (or alternatively masquerade as

ordinary consumers to do so), promoting particular brands or products.
(Discussions of these and other emerging strategies in marketing to children may be found in Calvert, 2003; Chung and Grimes, 2005; Grimes and Shade, 2005; Lindstrom and Seybold, 2003; Montgomery, 2007; Montgomery and Chester, 2009; and Wasko, 2010.)

As we saw in chapter 4, historical accounts such as those of Lisa Jacobson (2004) suggest that some of these more 'participatory' approaches are far from new, even if they are now operating on a very different scale. While they have attracted growing attention – and indeed considerable alarm among critics of marketing to children (e.g. Linn, 2004; Schor, 2004) – it is also important to recognize that more traditional forms of marketing have not been abandoned. Watching television is still far and away children's major leisure-time pursuit, and while television advertising generally is in decline (it was outpaced by online marketing in the UK in 2009), it remains a significant focus of expenditure.

These new techniques are fairly diverse, and some may ultimately prove much more successful than others – although the expenditure on such approaches is undoubtedly increasing quite significantly at present. However, they have certain qualities in common. For the most part, they are about *branding* – creating a set of values or emotions associated with the brand – rather than the marketing of specific products. Many of them depend to a large extent on the use of *digital media*, with its immediacy of access, its networking capacity, and its apparent 'youth' appeal, as well as its capacity for surveillance of consumer behaviour. Many are *'personalized'*, in the sense that they seem to appeal and respond to the individual's wants and needs, rather than addressing them as a member of a mass market. They are often *deceptive* or 'stealthy', in the sense that their persuasive intentions are not made apparent – for example through commercial messages being embedded in other content, rather than clearly identifiable as in the case of television commercials or banner advertising online. Finally, many of them are *'participatory'* or 'interactive', in that they require the positive involvement of the consumer, who may be called upon to engage actively with the communication, to pass it on to others, or even to help create the message. In this sense, they again reflect much broader trends in contemporary marketing, which seek to engage with individuals' sense of personal agency, and to create more intense forms of intimacy and 'bonding' in the relations between consumers and brands (Arvidsson, 2006).

The use of these innovative techniques raises important new questions about the ethics of marketing to children, and about children's understanding of commercial motivations and practices. Many of them blur the boundaries between promotional messages and other content, making it possible to embed advertising in contexts where it is less likely to be recognized as such. They often entail the gathering, aggregation and use of personal data about consumers without them necessarily being aware that this is taking place; and children may also be encouraged or required to provide personal information about others, for example parents or friends, without their knowledge, raising significant concerns about privacy (see Buckingham et al., 2007; Livingstone, 2006a; Nairn and Monkgol, 2007). 'Peer-to-peer' and viral marketing represent a modern form of 'word-of-mouth', although they also depend on a degree of deception, whereby users (rather than companies) are seen as the authors or at least the distributors of commercial messages. There are also justified concerns that children are being recruited for market research at an ever-younger age, and that the aims of such research are not always clearly explained. There may be further violations of privacy here, as such researchers are increasingly keen on studying children in their 'natural habitat' of the home or the peer group. Finally, there are questions about who owns the 'user-generated' material that children supply in this context: children's blogs, their contributions to chatrooms or social networking sites, or the photographs or videos they post on sharing sites may in fact be owned by the proprietors of those sites, who may be able to sell this material on. In all these respects, it could well be argued that the 'terms of trade' of such practices are not always sufficiently well explained, or indeed observed.

As we have seen in chapter 4, a fair amount is known about children's understanding of television advertising, although the research remains contested in some respects. However, relatively little is known about how they engage with the commercial messages and tactics used in newer media. Underlying these debates are continuing questions about the level and nature of children's *competence* as consumers, and the relationship between competence and actual behaviour. For example, children are generally believed to be capable of understanding the persuasive intentions of a television advertisement from the age of 7 or 8; but does that understanding necessarily transfer to practices such as product placement, embedded advertising or viral marketing? Indeed, to what extent do most *adults* recognize the commercial nature and persuasive intentions of such practices? And even if they do, to what extent is this kind of 'digital literacy' necessarily a useful defence against persuasion?

The few existing studies in this area have identified some justified ethical concerns about company practices, but there is much less reliable evidence about how consumers understand or respond to them. A recent UK study found that children were generally aware of (and resistant towards) online advertising and marketing 'scams', although they were less aware of 'stealthy' techniques such as advergames and product placement, and the commercial dimensions of the internet more broadly (Fiedler et al., 2007; Nairn and Dew, 2007). While parents seemed very aware of safety and privacy issues, they were less aware of (and much less concerned about) the commercial dimensions, although both parents and children appeared to have learnt from the mistakes they had made in this respect. Yet, given that promotional messages are now more invisibly embedded in other content, it seems likely that understanding persuasive intent will be a much more complex matter; and it is reasonable to assume that children (and adults) are less likely to understand the commercial dimensions of online marketing than those of 'older' media.

However, in some respects the issues raised here go beyond questions about children's competence, or lack of it. Children (or indeed adults) may be more or less knowledgeable about such techniques, but that knowledge in itself does not necessarily confer the power to resist them. Likewise, the fact that children are now increasingly addressed and engaged as 'active' consumers does not necessarily mean that they have greater agency. Taken together, these developments might be seen to represent a paradigm shift in the nature of marketing, away from a 'mass marketing' model to one that is significantly more pervasive, more personalized and more participatory. In this context, consumers' agency itself is being produced and engaged in new ways, which require us to move beyond the dichotomous thinking that so frequently characterizes discussions of children's consumer culture.

Conclusion

Like the previous one, this chapter has focused rather more on the ideas and practices of marketers than of children themselves. The self-evident problem with this approach is that it may end up implicitly according greater power to marketers than they in fact possess. As I have suggested, contemporary marketing is an increasingly uncertain and risky process, in which success (that is, profit) is very far from guaranteed. Marketers attempt to understand and control consumers, but consumers do not always behave in expected or well-disciplined ways. This may be particularly the case with children, who are a comparatively fast-moving, volatile market. Yet while we need to avoid the temptation to mythologize marketers as evil manipulators of the innocent, we also need to avoid the equivalent temptation with children. Children do enjoy a degree of power and agency in their dealings with the market: they can and do resist what they are offered, and they can appropriate and use it in diverse and unpredictable ways. However, that power is very far from absolute: children have relatively little say in determining the range of products – and hence of meanings and pleasures – that the market makes available to them. Yet the issue here is not so much one of relative *degrees* of power. Rather, as I have attempted to show in this chapter, the power relationships between marketers and children are jointly constructed by both parties. The paradox of contemporary marketing – both to children and to adults – is that it increasingly requires and depends upon an 'active' consumer.

6

The fear of fat

Obesity, food and consumption

In 2007, the British media regulator Ofcom (the Office of Communications) began to implement new restrictions on the television advertising of food and drink products to children. The measures impose a total ban on the advertising of food and drink that is high in fat, salt and sugar (HFSS) in and around programmes with particular appeal to children under the age of 16; along with additional rules on the content of advertisements aimed specifically at children of primary school age (for example, prohibiting the use of celebrities and licensed characters). Ofcom estimated that these measures would result in children under 16 being exposed to 41 per cent fewer advertisements for HFSS products, while, for children under 9, the reduction would be 51 per cent (Ofcom, 2006). Subsequent monitoring suggested that, while there was a reduction, these targets were unduly optimistic, although children's exposure to such advertising (and overall expenditure on television advertising) had apparently been falling in any case prior to the restrictions being introduced (Department of Health, 2008; Ofcom, 2008a, b).

The new regulations were explicitly defined by Ofcom as a contribution to the British government's ongoing attempts to reduce childhood obesity (Ofcom, 2007a). Yet, while it had been clearly foreshadowed in the Department of Health White Paper *Choosing Health*, published in 2004, Ofcom's move went further than many observers had expected – although some campaigners have continued to complain that it has not gone far enough. It was also somewhat at odds with its own position some years earlier, when it had seemed generally wary of increasing regulation in this area (Ofcom, 2004). These new measures are stricter than those in nearly all other industrialized countries: even Sweden, which has a complete ban on advertising to children (at least on terrestrial channels), places the cut-off point at the age of 12.

This chapter sets out to provide a broad view of the debate about children's food consumption, and particularly about the role of advertising and marketing. I begin by considering the recent wave of concern around childhood obesity, which has arguably now reached the status of a new 'moral panic'. I then look more specifically at the impact of advertising and marketing, and the evidence from research. This research – like other forms of media effects research – tends to isolate children's consumption from the wider social context, and from the many other factors that influence both food consumption and the incidence of obesity itself. In the later sections of the chapter, I therefore seek to outline an alternative approach, drawing both on sociological and anthropological research into children's and families' consumption of food, and on analyses of the political economy of food production and distribution.

The making of the 'obesity epidemic'

The claim that obesity has now reached 'epidemic' proportions is routinely rehearsed in the public debate. As well as reducing overall wellbeing and quality of life, obesity is deemed to be a significant cause of a range of potentially fatal illnesses, including cancer, heart disease and Type 2 diabetes. Levels of childhood obesity, we are told, have risen precipitously; and when these increases are projected over the coming decades, the resulting pressure on the health service and the economy will be impossible to sustain. This generation of children will apparently be the first to have lower life expectancy than their parents.

These issues have become the focus of an avalanche of media coverage. Alarming accounts of children 'dying' from obesity, of obesity as the new 'Black Death', and of the obesity 'timebomb' regularly hit the headlines. TV documentaries feature children sent to 'fat camps' and subjected to healthy eating regimes in schools, while 'obesity scientists' speculate about the dire long-term consequences for health of fast-food diets. Such assertions are reinforced by the pronouncements of government representatives – including the US Surgeon General, who has claimed that obesity is 'a greater threat than weapons of mass destruction'.[1] (For further instances, see Basham et al., 2006; Evans et al., 2008b; Julier, 2008.)

Critics of such 'obesity discourse' suggest that the evidence for these claims is very limited. Clearly, obesity is not a communicable disease, and as such cannot be regarded as an 'epidemic' (a term routinely used in this context by the UK government's former Chief Medical Officer, Sir Liam Donaldson). BMI (Body Mass Index), which is typically used as a measure of overweight and obesity, is both arbitrary and misleading, not least because it assesses body mass rather than fat. The thresholds for the categories of overweight and obesity have been lowered in recent years, and much of the public discussion conflates the two categories, resulting in very high proportions of people being defined as 'overweight-and-obese'. Critics also challenge the claim that childhood obesity is rising significantly, and dispute the validity of long-term projections.[2]

More broadly, critics argue that the links between obesity and diet, and between obesity and disease or premature death, are not straightforward. While there has been an overall historical trend towards a small weight gain over the past century, this can be seen as a general consequence of better nutrition, food quality and safety, and rising standards of living (which have also resulted in gains in average height, for example). Over the same period, there have also been significant increases in longevity. Although the small minority of 'morbidly' obese people has grown, the rise in average weight among the population as a whole has been of the order of a few pounds (Evans et al., 2008b). Children's ingestion of calories has actually declined – although their amount of physical activity and energy expenditure has declined more quickly. However, obesity is not simply a matter of the balance between 'energy in' and 'energy out', but is also subject to a range of other environmental and genetic factors: there is no clear causal relationship between increased intake of calories or dietary fat and levels of adiposity. Despite the widespread use of BMI, good health cannot simply be equated with thinness or with a lower body mass (Critical analysis of the data on such issues can be found in Basham et al., 2006; Campos, 2004; Gard and Wright, 2005; Monaghan, 2007; and Social Issues Research Centre (SIRC), 2005.)

The contemporary concern about childhood obesity has been strongly fuelled by the public relations activities of the weight-loss and pharmaceutical industries, which have sponsored a good deal of the research and played a key role in political lobbying on the issue – as well as the insurance industry, which has much to gain from the creation of new categories of risk. The result, as Basham et al. (2006) suggest, has been a systematic manipulation and misrepresentation of the scientific evidence. As with the debate about 'toxic childhood', we can identify key claims-makers – 'obesity entrepreneurs' – who are actively using the media to orchestrate the campaign and to marginalize dissenting views, thereby encouraging the impression that there is a scientific consensus (see also Julier, 2008). Meanwhile, the expert 'medicalization' of obesity – its official recognition as a disease, and hence as a focus for medical intervention – clearly works to the benefit of the medical profession, along with the drug and diet industries.

Here again, while other age groups may be equally, if not more, prone to obesity, the specific focus on children provides a powerful means of mobilizing concern and commanding assent – and indeed of justifying forms of regulation that might otherwise be seen as unacceptable. As Evans et al. (2008b) suggest, obesity has become the focus of a 'latter day child saving movement', which employs a familiar rhetoric of child abuse and protection. As Tingstad (2009) argues, there is an 'interdependence of panics' here, as concerns about childhood obesity both reinforce and are reinforced by other concerns about the apparent demise of traditional notions of childhood.

However, the characterization of the issue as a 'moral panic' tends to imply that it is merely an irrational phenomenon – a temporary form of madness. Others have argued that the contemporary preoccupation with obesity is more profound, and indeed indicative of much broader social and historical trends (see Beardsworth and Keil, 1998; Evans et al., 2008b). Historically, standards of beauty and attractiveness – and indeed of physical health – have been highly variable. In earlier centuries, body fat was often seen as an indication of social status; and desirable body shapes (as featured, for example, in the visual arts) were significantly more ample than those in today's media. As recently as the early decades of the twentieth century, the key health concern as regards the poor was not with obesity but with undernourishment. Our current preoccupation with the need to be slim – and the extensive forms of work and expenditure that it can often entail – is a relatively recent phenomenon.

As Alan Beardsworth and Teresa Keil (1998) have pointed out, there are some interesting paradoxes here. In modern industrialized societies, food is mostly plentiful but growing numbers of people are following restricted diets. Body weight is slightly increasing, yet the desirable body image promoted in the media has arguably become slimmer. Obesity may be rising, but so too are eating disorders such as anorexia and bulimia. As these and other authors suggest, our contemporary preoccupation with slim bodies reflects a broader emphasis on self-regulation and self-discipline that is characteristic of the governance of 'late modern' societies (see also Evans et al., 2008b). Particularly for young women, the possession of a slim body is often perceived as a symbol of personal success in the competitive environment of the modern economy (Harris, 2004a). This preoccupation also feeds a range of other commercial enterprises, including the slimming, health food and fitness industries, and the media that are associated with them. Fat is highly profitable, as the proliferation of patented diet regimes, weight loss treatments, fitness products and slimming 'superfoods' amply demonstrates.

None of this is to imply that the rise in obesity is merely an illusion – although it is to suggest that the scale and severity of the problem has been overstated. 'Morbid' obesity does represent a significant health risk, and it has certainly increased, although it remains a comparatively rare condition. More significantly, the tendency to present obesity as an individual (and indeed moral) failing tends to obscure the social and cultural factors that are in play. At least in industrialized countries, poor people are more likely to be obese than wealthy people, as are those in particular non-white ethnic groups (see Julier, 2008; Patel, 2007; Wang and Lobstein, 2006), but the neglect of such factors results in a situation where such people are seen to be solely responsible for their fate, and become prime targets for greater surveillance and regulation (Julier, 2008).

These issues will be discussed a little more fully in the conclusion of this chapter; although it should be noted that there is something of a tension here between the tendency to blame the individual and the tendency to blame the media, and specifically advertising (see Tingstad, 2009). It is to this latter issue that we turn in the following section.

Advertising, obesity and the problem of evidence

As with the construction of the 'obesity epidemic' itself, there are considerable grounds for scepticism about the arguments that are typically made about marketing and advertising in this respect. In an earlier analysis (Buckingham, 2009a, b), I have explored some of the ways in which research evidence was used by the various contending participants in the debate about food advertising and children in the years leading up to Ofcom's decision. Despite some claims that there is an emerging consensus here, reviews of the research disagree – in some cases, quite profoundly – in their overall conclusions. Key reviews commissioned by bodies such as the UK Ministry of Agriculture, Fisheries and Food (Young et al., 1996), the Food Standards Agency (Hastings et al., 2003), the Advertising Association (Young, 2003), Ofcom (Livingstone, 2004, 2006b; Livingstone and Helsper, 2004) and the US Institute of Medicine (McGinnis et al., 2006) tend to tell conflicting or inconsistent stories. The various parties involved have also commissioned further reviews that seek to discredit their opponents' arguments, in each case appealing to the apparent objectivity of scientific evidence (see Buckingham, 2009a). While the reviews themselves are mostly careful and qualified, the conclusions contained in their executive summaries are sometimes quite different, and in some instances they have also been 'spun' in press releases in rather misleading ways (see Ambler, 2006).

Despite the apparent insistence on 'evidence-based policy' that is characteristic of contemporary government, there would seem to be a significant mismatch here between the policy that finally appeared and the evidence that was adduced to support it. Following two commissioned reviews, Ofcom's initial response was relatively cautious, suggesting that the available evidence was limited; and it appeared to be leaning against additional regulation, not least on the grounds that it was unlikely to be effective (Ofcom, 2004). Tessa Jowell, then Minister for Culture, Media and Sport, seemed to agree (as cited in Basham et al., 2006: 213). However, as political pressure mounted following its public consultation, Ofcom appeared to change its view, referring specifically to the 'significant body of available research' justifying the move (Ofcom, 2007a). In fact, as I shall indicate below, the research it cited here, the US Institute of Medicine review (McGinnis et al., 2006), does not justify such a decision – nor, indeed, do the conclusions of its own reviews.

This dubious use of research evidence is by no means unprecedented in the field of media policy: indeed, Willard Rowland's 25-year-old study of *The Politics of TV Violence* (1983) traces very similar processes in the debates around television violence in the 1960s and 1970s. Rowland describes how the broadcasting industry and government policy-makers funded and subsequently used research in their attempts to define (or redefine) social issues for their own purposes. Rowland's key point is that the focus on the effects of television violence – and the small reprimands and marginal changes in regulation that resulted from it – enabled both government and the industry to deflect attention away from much broader concerns to do with the social and cultural functions of television, and indeed from the wider causes of violence in society. The perpetually inconclusive or qualified findings of effects research legitimized both parties' attempts to avoid fundamental changes in communications policy that might have upset the commercial status quo – while simultaneously allowing them to appear responsible, and as though they were responding to public concern.

In this case, my analysis suggests that, despite the appeal to scientific evidence, the decision to ban HFSS food advertising was politically driven: the government needed to be seen to be 'doing something' about the problem of child obesity, and regulating advertising provided a high-profile and comparatively easy way of achieving this. As I have noted above, the new restrictions have resulted in a reduction in children's exposure to HFSS advertising, at least on children's television, although such a reduction was occurring in any case.[3] Whether or not they have succeeded in reducing levels of child obesity remains to be demonstrated – although it would probably be impossible to show this in any case. Certainly, countries that have banned advertising to children – such as Sweden, Norway, Greece and the Canadian province of Quebec – do not appear to have done so: in all these countries, child obesity has actually risen in recent years in line with global trends (Basham et al., 2006; Tingstad, 2009).

Meanwhile, there have been other, more counter-productive consequences. The advertising of full-fat milk, cheese and nuts to children is now prohibited on the grounds of their fat content. More seriously, children's commercial TV producers have used the loss of advertising revenue to justify a significant reduction in domestically produced programming for children (PACT, 2006) – although this too was in decline in any case, as Ofcom's own research suggests (Ofcom, 2007b; and see chapter 11). More broadly, there is a risk that the regulation of advertising will be regarded as a substitute for the more far-reaching and complex measures that may be required, for example in order to address the well-established connections between obesity and child poverty.

As research has (not) shown ...

So what does the research on this issue actually prove? To start with, it does demonstrate fairly clearly that most television food advertising is indeed for HFSS food. Prior to the recent restrictions, in 2004 Ofcom estimated the total UK advertising spend per annum in the categories of food, soft drinks and chain restaurants as £742 million, with £522 million spent on television advertising – although only £32 million of this was spent in children's airtime. Food advertising on television was found to be dominated by breakfast cereals, confectionery, savoury snacks and soft drinks, with fast-food restaurants making a more recent entry into the market, while advertising for staple items and fresh foods was declining. Although (as I have noted), the new regulations have eliminated such advertising during children's programming, children do, of course, continue to be exposed to mainstream programmes, and the balance here is likely to remain fairly similar.

However, when it comes to assessing the influence of such advertising, the evidence is much less clear. It should be noted at the outset here that the vast bulk of this research is about television advertising, rather than other aspects of marketing; and about food preference rather than other potential causes of obesity. Much of the research is also relatively old, and most of it was undertaken in the United States – factors which limit its wider relevance to the contemporary situation in the UK or elsewhere. Most of this work derives from the mainstream media effects research tradition: it conceives of the relationship between messages and receivers as one of stimulus and response, and tends to represent children in particular as passive and incompetent viewers (see chapter 3).

Of course, there is little doubt that television advertising can be effective, in the sense that it can influence people to buy things; and, given that most food advertising is for HFSS foods, it seems fairly logical to suggest that it is likely at least to contribute to the prevalence of 'less healthy' diets among children.[4] Advertisers, however, frequently argue that the influence of advertising is primarily confined to brand preference rather than category preference – that is, for one brand rather than another, not one type of food rather than another. Advertising may encourage us to eat Burger King rather than McDonalds, but not more hamburgers and less broccoli. However, this is a contested point: critics of HFSS advertising argue that advertising influences children in both respects. Even so, few studies in this area make sufficient distinctions between brand awareness, brand preference, brand consumption and category consumption.

While there has been a fair amount of research on the relationship between the advertising and consumption of food, not all of it is directly relevant to the question of obesity. Research has generally explored food preference, or at best food choice (often under artificial conditions), rather than obesity per se. However, the relationship between the food people say they prefer and what they actually eat is not straightforward. They are not always able to eat what they would ideally wish to eat: a whole range of other factors, most notably price and availability, come into play. As such, an expressed preference for 'unhealthy' foods among children cannot on its own be taken to result in (or be equated with) obesity. Furthermore, it appears that taste preferences and dietary patterns are largely determined by other factors, and are in place from a very young age, well before children become aware of advertising. The early years are especially important: once established, taste preferences and eating habits appear to continue with relatively little change for the rest of a person's life (see Young, 2003).

Food consumption is, of course, only one contributory factor in obesity. Some people are more genetically disposed towards obesity, or have an inherited preference for sweet food. Aspects of family interaction also play a role: obese children are more likely to have obese or overweight parents, although children may well ask for many things that (for a variety of reasons) they do not get. Lifestyle, and particularly the amount of physical exercise people take, is another key factor. As I have noted, children's calorie intake has in fact slightly declined, although there has been an increase in dietary fat intake as a proportion of overall diet (Prentice and

Jebb, 1995). However, the number of calories they burn through exercise has declined more quickly (Barwise et al., 2009; Basham et al., 2006). This may relate to a number of other factors, not least the decline in free access to public space for play (see chapter 11).

This research also suffers from some familiar methodological problems, of the kind discussed in chapter 3. A particular problem here relates to the ways in which children's exposure to advertising is measured. In most cases, what researchers measure is in fact the total amount of television viewing (often as estimated by parents). But the total amount of television people watch is not necessarily a reliable measure of their exposure to advertising, especially if there are channels (as in the UK) that do not carry advertising. Meanwhile, other research has suggested that television programming more generally is dominated by instances of people eating 'healthy' food such as fruit and vegetables (Dickinson, 2000; Oates, 2009) – which would further suggest that it is vital to differentiate between viewing in general and the viewing of advertising in particular.

There are also many possible ways in which television viewing might be associated with obesity. Watching television is a sedentary activity, which does not burn a great many calories. People who watch a lot of television (or indeed, read a lot of books) tend to do less exercise, and are more likely to prefer other sedentary activities. People tend to snack while they watch television, and may be less inclined to stop when they are full. Television is also a relatively inexpensive form of entertainment, which is a major reason why it is more heavily watched in less wealthy families, who are also more likely to be obese. Here again, it is very difficult to establish evidence of the *causal* role of advertising. It may be that advertising encourages people to eat an unhealthy diet, which in turn is one contributory factor in obesity. But it may equally be that people who are disposed (for various reasons) to eat an unhealthy diet – or are unable to afford a healthy one – are also inclined to watch a lot of television.

So to what extent does advertising (or marketing more broadly) contribute to childhood obesity? It seems reasonable to conclude that advertising does have an impact, but the research is frustratingly limited and inconclusive. While there is a large volume of work in the general area, there is actually very little that is both *directly relevant* – in the sense that it focuses specifically on exposure to advertising, and on the effects on obesity – and *reliable* – in that it addresses some of the more obvious methodological limitations. Despite their differences, most reviews of the research agree that the impact, if any, is small. One frequently quoted figure is that exposure to television advertising accounts for some 2 per cent of the variation in children's food choice (a figure that comes from a study by Bolton (1983), which found that parents were fifteen times more important than advertising as an influence on children's eating). It should be noted that food choice is only one factor in obesity, and, as such, the influence on obesity is bound to be even smaller than this; although one could argue that a variation of 2 per cent is nevertheless significant across the population as a whole. Even so, we have very little definitive evidence on the relative size of any such effect, or how it might interact with other factors.

The most recent systematic review in this area was produced by the US Institute of Medicine (McGinnis et al., 2006). This report concludes that there is strong evidence that television advertising influences the food and beverage preferences, purchasing requests and beliefs of younger children (aged 2-11), although the evidence on those aged 12-18 is deemed to be insufficient. Even so, the ultimate conclusion of the report is that there is insufficient evidence to establish a causal relationship between the viewing of television advertising and adiposity; and it also says little about the *relative importance* of different factors in the development of obesity (see Barwise et al., 2009). Interestingly, however, this review was 'spun' in the media as providing definitive evidence of the harmful influence of advertising (see Basham et al., 2006); and, as I have noted, it was specifically cited by Ofcom as grounds for what appeared to be a significant change in their view on the issue, and hence for introducing new regulations.

Finally, it should be emphasized here that most of this research relates only to television advertising – which, as we have seen, is only part of the broader marketing environment. Point-of-sale displays, sponsorship, media tie-ins and product placement are all widely used in food marketing. One apparent consequence of the new regulations on television advertising in the UK is that marketers have been encouraged to divert their efforts online (although this was happening in any case). Recent research has drawn attention to some of the strategies that are being adopted by food marketers in this context – which include branded environments, advergames, mobile and viral marketing, and behavioural profiling (see Montgomery and Chester, 2007, 2009). Of course, these other forms of promotion might well be seen to amplify the effects of television advertising, although (as I have noted in chapter 5) very little is known about how children respond to them, and the effects they may have.

Advertising in context

Ultimately, the key problem with the research in this field is that it tends to consider the relationship between marketing and obesity (or rather, in most cases, television advertising and food preference) in isolation from other social factors, or to account for these other factors in unduly simplified ways. Basham et al. (2006) present an indicative list of no fewer than thirty-nine 'risk factors' that have been shown or hypothesized to play a role in obesity, ranging from birth weight, parental adiposity, gender, social class and race, through to levels of physical activity, eating habits and preferences, and use of media. As they argue, most of the studies that purport to identify the influence of advertising have failed to control for even a handful of these factors.

In my view, this points to the need for a more comprehensive socio-cultural analysis of children's food consumption. Such an analysis would need to address everyday consumption practices – the purchasing, preparation and 'provisioning' of food, the social relationships that surround it, and the meanings and pleasures that attach to it. It would also need to address a wider range of economic factors that relate to the production and distribution of food. While marketing would play a part in such an analysis, it is also important to take account of pricing, as well as the availability of particular types of food in local communities, which may represent an important constraint on diets, especially in low-income families. In the following sections, I discuss some research that addresses the kinds of issues that have been raised here.

Understanding children's food cultures

Food is self-evidently both a material and a cultural phenomenon. There are significant social, historical and cultural variations in what people eat and how they eat it. Food itself is invested with values, emotions and symbolic meanings, which enable us to distinguish between what is edible and inedible, healthy and unhealthy, high status and low status, and so on. Meanwhile, the ways in which food is prepared, served and eaten also help to construct social relationships, and to demonstrate forms of intimacy and care, as well as social power and authority. There have been numerous sociological and anthropological studies of these different aspects of 'food culture', ranging from structuralist analyses of the symbolic 'grammar' of food classification to more culturalist accounts of the consumption and use of food in everyday life (see, for example, Ashley et al., 2004; Beardsworth and Keil, 1998; Warde, 1997).

Thus, historical research has considered the changing nature both of diets themselves and of eating practices (food etiquette or 'table manners'). Stephen Mennell (1985), for example, traces the gradual 'civilizing' of appetite in England and France since the Middle Ages: he describes how authorities such as the state, the church and the medical establishment encouraged populations to internalize constraints on the expression of appetite, and to maintain public decorum while eating. Other studies have focused on the ways in which the provisioning, marketing and consumption of food acts as a marker of particular ethnic or national identities (Ashley et al., 2004). In the contemporary context, research has also focused on the *mediation* of food, for example in cookbooks, television shows and news media – which, of course, play a key role in defining nutritional beliefs and standards, and in shaping consumption practices (e.g. Hollows, 2003; Warde, 1997).

Here again, consumption must be seen not simply as a matter of what we *do* with goods, but with what they *say* (cf. Douglas and Isherwood, 1979). Taste in food serves as a means of performing or expressing particular identities (defined, for example, in terms of social class, ethnicity, gender and age) and of articulating social life. Bourdieu's notion of cultural capital (introduced in chapter 2) has obvious applications to the study of food cultures (Bourdieu, 1979). Food itself – and the practices that surround it – can actively symbolize and mark out social and cultural distinctions, although the food choices of particular social groups also *reflect* the wider inequalities that are at stake in such a process (Beardsworth and Keil, 1998).

In the case of children, the dimension of power and inequality is often very apparent. The notion that children (other than babies) should have different food from adults appears to be a relatively recent development, and is far from universal. According to Mennell (1985), this idea arose in Victorian England in the context of wider changes in beliefs about child rearing. At least in Britain, the key characteristic of children's food was that it be plain and bland; and, as Corrigan (1997: 121-3) suggests, this might be seen as a further means of disciplining children – developing the sensuality of the palate might have been seen as opening the door to other unacceptable aspects of sensuality as well. Corrigan argues that training children to enjoy food that adults deem to be 'good for them' is itself very likely to produce 'faddy' or 'picky' eating; and, as children get older, they may tend to avoid foods that are associated with younger children.

Meanwhile, sociological and anthropological studies point to the crucial role of meals in *producing* family relationships, and indeed the idea of family itself. For example, the 'proper family dinner' is often taken as a key symbol of family togetherness – although it is also a relatively recent practice, dating back only to the mid nineteenth century. The 'proper dinner' enacts power relationships based on gender as well as age, not least because it is most frequently mothers who cook (de Vault, 1991; Warde, 1997). However, Allison James and her colleagues (2009) suggest that this process varies according to the different 'generational order' of families – that is, the extent to which children are perceived as more or less autonomous or dependent. In the British families they studied, different eating practices reflected different ways of 'doing family' and different levels of participation on the part of children. In some instances, a more egalitarian generational order was reflected in a shared approach to preparing food; while in others, the 'proper dinner' was still very much seen as an index of the mother's care. However, food and eating did not always bear this symbolic significance: as James et al. suggest, food may not always be the main medium through which family togetherness and identification are expressed.

By contrast, Dan Cook (2009a, b) sees this in rather more stark terms, as an ongoing power struggle between mothers on the one hand, and children and marketers on the other. As Cook suggests, the struggle here is largely about the social *meaning* of food – that is, about how particular foods and eating occasions are defined and categorized (for example, as healthy or unhealthy, as meals or snacks, as treats or staple items), and about how such distinctions are blurred or maintained. In the course of this 'semantic labour', mothers adopt a range of strategies, from compromise and bargaining through rules and reward systems to deception and outright coercion. As Cook suggests, the child often has a considerable degree of agency in this process – although this agency is largely aligned with (and some would say exploited by) the market. While the mother's attempts to impose a particular 'alimentary order' may be disrupted by circumstances, as well as by peers and (on occasion) more pliable fathers, it is 'incessant' commercial marketing that constitutes the most significant force to be reckoned with.

Of course, it is generally parents who purchase food, even if they subsequently have to struggle to persuade their children to eat it. Other studies suggest that parents still have a considerable degree of power to determine what children eat, and that many children have internalized parental prescriptions about 'healthy eating' – albeit sometimes more at the level of aspiration or self-justification than actual practice (Dryden et al., 2009; Evans et al., 2008b; Marshall et al., 2007). Such studies suggest that stories of parents being subjected to 'pester power' induced by advertising are somewhat oversimplified; and that children are in fact often resistant to the appeals of brands and licensed characters. However, food manufacturers and marketers are bound to find ways of addressing this ambivalence and negotiation. Albeit more in some cultures than others, particular items are commercially demarcated as 'children's food', but they are also designed to appeal to parents as well. Thus, the marketing of so-called 'fun food' typically emphasizes nutritional value (often in the form of added 'healthy' elements), while also seeking to accentuate the entertainment potential of food, for example in the use of particular shapes and colours, as well as licensed characters and other media tie-ins. As Dryden et al. (2009) suggest, this tension between individual agency and choice on the one hand, and moral imperatives to do with 'healthy eating' on the other, is characteristic of contemporary food cultures more broadly, not only in relation to children (cf. Warde, 1997).

The other side of the story, however, is to do with what children choose to consume when they are beyond the reach of parental surveillance. Allison James's (1982) study of children's consumption of sweets (candy) is a particular case in point here. James explores the taste of children in the North of England for a particular form of inexpensive confectionery that they refer to as 'kets' – a word that in adult talk is equivalent to 'rubbish'. According to James, these sweets are defined not only by their cheapness, but also by their contrast with adult notions of acceptable food (including adult confectionery). This is apparent not only in their physical qualities – they typically have bright primary colours, artificial flavours and fantastical shapes – but also in the ways in which they are bought and shared, often with little attention to hygiene. James suggests that kets represent a conscious violation of the normal eating conventions of adult society: they belong to the 'disorderly and inverted world of children', and represent a kind of temporary 'carnivalesque' subversion of the dominant generational order. While kets are a specific 'local' example, they clearly exemplify a broader ambivalence around the symbolism of sugar and sweetness – as something 'naughty but nice' – which is again characteristic of contemporary food cultures more generally, including those of adults (see Beardsworth and Keil, 1998: ch. 11).[5]

These accounts reflect the ways in which the provision and consumption of food for children are tied up with the creation of a generational order – that is, with the mutual construction of identities by adults and children. In the term proposed by Leena Alanen (2001), this is an instance of 'generationing', of the *performance* of generationally defined identities (see chapter 3). Parents' provision of food for their children is about enacting relationships of care and intimacy, but also about imposing a structure of power and authority – and, as such, it is perhaps bound to meet with resistance.

The food system

In addition to analysing 'food cultures', there is also a need to understand the food *system*, or the political economy of food. Here again, there have been significant historical and cultural variations in the ways in which food is produced, distributed and consumed. The modern food system has been transformed through the use of industrialized, large-scale production methods, new techniques of preservation, processing and transportation, and changing practices in terms of packaging, marketing, retailing and food service (for example in restaurants). This is an increasingly globalized market, which has been made possible by the deregulation of trade and neo-liberal 'free-market' policies – although large transnational companies are also struggling to adapt to 'local' needs. The food business has seen a significant concentration of ownership, with growing numbers of mergers and acquisitions, especially in the distribution and retail sectors. Meanwhile, small farmers are very much at the bottom of the pile: it has become more and more difficult for farmers in developing countries to earn a living, and they suffer from increasing insecurity and exploitative working conditions. (For accounts of these developments, see Beardsworth and Keil, 1998; Lang and Heasman, 2004; and Patel, 2007.)

These developments present significant and growing challenges for environmental sustainability, which are to some extent accentuated by the use of Genetic Modification (GM) technologies. Although the food system appears to be increasingly rationalized, it is also prone to crisis, as the rising incidence of health and safety scares illustrates. These developments also raise concerns about global inequalities, both at an individual and a national level, as the food system is increasingly implicated in 'structural readjustment programmes' and debt regimes that operate to the benefit of Western countries. While the industrialized nations can be accused of over-consumption, developing countries suffer from under-consumption. Although diet-related conditions such as obesity and diabetes are increasing worldwide, and heart disease is also increasing in the developing world, mass hunger persists (Lang and Heasman, 2004).

One aspect that is particularly relevant here is the change in patterns of food distribution and retailing. As I have noted, there has been growing concentration of ownership in the retail sector, with large supermarkets exercising increasing power over the entire food supply chain (a tendency that is especially pronounced in the UK). From the point of view of the consumer, our massive out-of-town supermarkets might be seen as the ultimate fulfilment of consumer choice, although they also represent the triumph of 'scientific management', in terms of their ability to regulate consumer behaviour, and to gather data about individual consumers (most notably through 'loyalty card' schemes). Critics frequently attack supermarket chains for price fixing and profiteering, exploitative labour practices, the destruction of local communities and the squeezing out of competition. However, one less easily recognized aspect of changes in food retailing has been the 'redlining' of poorer neighbourhoods, and the phenomenon of 'food deserts'. In some areas, it is hard to access food shops without a car; poor people may have to pay significantly more for food bought in neighbourhood stores; and as a result, they may have fewer options in terms of fresh or 'healthy' food – as well as having fewer opportunities for physical recreation (Patel, 2007: 241-3, 271-2).

A full exploration of these issues is obviously beyond the scope of this book. However, they do suggest that the representation of obesity as an *individual* problem – as a matter of personal morality, or as a medical issue – is at least an oversimplification. In spite of the rhetoric and appearance of greater choice, individuals have only a limited power to determine their own food consumption; and poor people in particular may find it especially difficult to afford and gain access to fresh fruit and vegetables, for example (Lang and Heasman, 2004: 252). One of the abiding reasons why many people eat so-called 'junk food' is because economies of scale make it relatively inexpensive to buy – and the provision of greater nutritional advice or the banning of television advertising is unlikely to make much difference to that. Yet despite their lack of choice, it would seem that individuals are increasingly called upon to take personal responsibility for what they eat.

The late modern diet

Taken together, these changes in food cultures and in the food system have had several implications for consumers (see Beardsworth and Keil, 1998; Lang and Heasman, 2004). At least in industrialized countries, we have fewer choices in terms of where to shop, but significantly greater diversity of products. The rise of out-of-town supermarkets has led to consumers spending greater amounts of time travelling to shops, but they are spending less time actually preparing meals. People are now more frequently eating out in restaurants – especially fast-food restaurants – and making use of 'convenience' foods, which often tend to be higher in fat, salt and sugar. 'Grazing' or snacking has become a commonplace mode of food consumption; and, while the 'proper family dinner' has by no means disappeared, it appears to be becoming a less frequent event. Of course, these developments also need to be seen in the light of other changes in family life, not least longer working hours, changing roles for women, and the increasing numbers of single-parent families, and families in which both parents are working (see chapter 8).

On the other hand, the industrialization of the food supply chain has led to rising concerns about food safety, and there has been growing resistance to the perceived 'corporate control' of food supply (Lang and Heasman, 2004). Yet, while 'food scares' of various kinds are widely circulated (see Ashley et al., 2004), safer or more 'ethical' alternatives – such as organic or 'natural' foods – are inevitably more expensive, and are much more likely to be taken up by wealthier groups.

However, Alan Warde's (1997) research, which is based on an extensive analysis of magazine articles about food as well as survey data about household consumption in the UK, suggests that changes in food practices have been less dramatic and more ambivalent than some have suggested. Warde identifies a series of tensions or 'antinomies' in contemporary food culture. The pressure towards innovation is set against the persistence (and reinvention) of tradition; the imperative of health is contrasted with the emphasis on indulgence; the need for economy is opposed to extravagance; and convenience is set against the value of care. Warde finds that there have been historical changes here – for example, towards a greater emphasis on convenience and on health in particular – but that consumers find it increasingly difficult to balance these different imperatives. People typically shuttle between these antinomies, rewarding themselves for 'healthy' eating by indulging in 'unhealthy' treats, or compensating for self-denial with moments of extravagance. In Warde's view, this uncertainty reflects a form of ambivalence and anxiety that is characteristic of 'late modernity'; and, as Beardsworth and Keil (1998) also suggest, the forms of certainty that were provided by traditional food cultures are no longer available, and the advice of experts (for example in the areas of food safety and health) is more and more open to dispute. In this climate, people are increasingly seen to be responsible for regulating and disciplining their own behaviour, yet the principles on which they might do so are often unclear or contradictory.

Warde (1997) confirms the claim that contemporary consumers have a much wider range of foodstuffs available to them – a development that he sees as a consequence of market commodification – but he questions whether this is resulting in greater diversity in terms of individual diets. His survey research and national statistics suggest that there are still clear contrasts between working-class and middle-class diets, and that there has been relatively little convergence between them, at least over the past half-century. This might be seen to confirm the cultural analysis, as proposed for example by Bourdieu (1979), that food is a key arena for the maintenance of class distinctions, and that middle-class taste in particular is characterized by an emphasis on sobriety, delicacy and refinement, and hence by a preference for 'healthy' options (see Beardsworth and Keil, 1998). However, it is important not to forget the material dimensions of this: as I have argued, people on low incomes are less likely to have opportunities to consume fresh or 'healthy' food, and the possibility of wastage means they may be unwilling to experiment with unfamiliar items. On the other hand, they may struggle to afford items that they perceive to be in the mainstream of contemporary food culture (which include branded and highly advertised items) in their attempts to avoid stigma and the perception of exclusion – an issue that may be particularly pertinent for children (p. 94).

The regulation of bodies

Setting the issue of obesity within this broader context points towards a rather different analysis. Critics of 'obesity discourse' argue that it can be seen as a contemporary manifestation of a long-running attempt to manage and modify the dietary habits of the 'lower orders' of society. As Ashley at al. (2004) suggest, this form of regulation has often drawn on scientific 'evidence' to assert the superiority of middle-class taste, and to present working-class diets as 'pathological and nutritionally inadequate'. In the early decades of the twentieth century, such regulation was focused largely on undernourishment – and was partly provoked by the need to have a workforce that could be ready for war. Yet in recent years, attention has shifted from under-consumption to over-consumption. According to Beardsworth and Keil (1998), the focus has also moved away from centralized regulation (for example through rationing and the state provision of free foods and supplements) towards self-regulation, and this has extended from the affluent elite to the population as a whole. People are routinely exhorted and 'educated' to control their diets, not least through the advice of scientific and medical experts – although these rationalized notions often come up against older cultural values and 'folk wisdom' about food, with the result that they have only an uneven influence on people's actual consumption habits.

To some extent, this process can be seen as indicative of a more general form of 'work on the self' – of self-surveillance and self-control – that is characteristic of 'late modernity' (e.g. Giddens, 1991; N. Rose, 1999). Possessing a disciplined, slim body is widely seen as an index of successful neo-liberal subjectivity. Equally, lacking such attributes is regarded as an individual failing–a matter of stupidity, laziness or downright irresponsibility. As Raj Patel (2007: 273) puts it, obesity is perceived to be the consequence of 'an inability to deal with the farrago of choices available to us, a deficit of impulse control'. From this perspective, the fat body is conceived in pathological terms, as abject, unclean and impure, and as evidence of a lack of self-care.

In the process, the social dimensions and causes of health problems are effectively ignored. As we shall see in more detail in chapter 7, some have argued that this is a pressure that applies particularly powerfully to women – leading some to regard it as a form of 'backlash' against feminism, or at least as a paradoxical consequence of changing roles for women. In the case of obesity, particular ethnic groups (such as African-Americans) have also been a key target for blame and for intervention. Ultimately, however, it is the social class dimension that is particularly apparent. According to Julier (2008), obesity discourse operates as a way of blaming the poor and increasing the status of the rich – not least those who both construct, and purport to be able to 'treat', the obesity problem. It removes attention from the structural causes of health inequalities, and from the potential responsibility of government, and effectively blames the victims: people who are already second-class citizens are now seen to be responsible for their own plight, and too slothful or ignorant to do anything about it.

However, as we have seen, it is children who are often the most prominent focus of concern here, and the most convenient targets for intervention. As Evans et al. (2008b) describe, the drive to eliminate child obesity has led to some intensive and invasive forms of regulation in schools, including the mandatory weighing and measuring of children, the public shaming of those judged overweight or obese, and the imposition of highly prescriptive forms of dietary instruction and correction. The diet and weight-loss industry has played a key role here, not least in the introduction of new techniques and strategies, from 'exergaming' and pedometers to skinfold measurement. Such initiatives may prove distressing for children, and particularly alienating for working-class parents, who perceive themselves to be blamed for their inadequate parenting skills (Schee, 2009).

Critics of these initiatives suggest that they may result in children experiencing high levels of dissatisfaction with their bodies, and making dangerous attempts to remedy this: dieting in order to lose weight is a significant health risk, which can ultimately result in eating disorders.

However, other research suggests that young people may be critical of, and more and more resistant towards, the moral imperatives that are increasingly urged upon them.[6] While they may be well aware of media discourses about 'ideal bodies' and popular morality tales about the perils of obesity, they can also be highly critical of media hyperbole and the business interests they perceive as underlying it. All this would suggest that highly didactic or evangelical approaches to health education are unlikely to be effective.

So, to return to the beginning of this chapter, what are the implications of these arguments in terms of public policy? To start with, it is important to get the issue in perspective. 'Morbid' obesity is indeed a medical problem, on which it would make good sense to focus the available resources; but, for the majority of the population, the health implications of being slightly overweight are probably negligible – not least given that the definition of 'overweight' itself has changed. More broadly, as Lang and Heasman (2004) suggest, the individualistic framing of questions about food and diet tends to result in individualistic solutions – for example to do with the provision of nutritional advice or food labelling for consumers – which have significant limitations. Providing dietary guidelines and labelling products is itself a contentious process, but even if a clear system could be agreed, it is unlikely that individuals would be consistent in following it – and in any case it presumes that people are always wise and rational consumers, who have complete control over their eating behaviour.

Banning food advertising to children is most unlikely to make any difference – and in the countries where it has been tried, it has manifestly failed. It is a largely symbolic move that could well prove counter-productive, in the sense that it might convey the mistaken impression that something significant is actually being done. The problems at stake here are more far-reaching and more intractable. The connections between food consumption and public health are complex, but they need to be considered in the light of the broader changes I have identified both in 'food cultures' and in the food system. The key issue here is that of social inequality – of people's unequal access both to food itself and to opportunities for physical exercise. Ultimately, rendering individuals responsible for broader social problems is unlikely to be effective – especially if the individuals who are targeted have a limited capacity to do anything about them.

7

Too much, too soon?

Marketing, media and the sexualization of girls

In recent years, there has been growing concern about the 'sexualization' of children, and particularly of girls. As with obesity, much of the debate here has focused on the effects of commercial marketing and media. Campaigners have drawn attention to the 'trickle down' of adult fashions into the children's market, for example in the form of revealing clothing for girls, along with items such as push-up bras, thongs, stilettos and 'saucy slogan' T-shirts. Media targeting young people – teen soaps, music videos and girls' magazines – have been accused of glamourizing casual sex and cultivating a 'throwaway' attitude to relationships. Teenagers have apparently become a lucrative market for the 'beauty industry', with growing amounts being spent on cosmetics, slimming products and plastic surgery. For younger children, the concern has focused on items such as make-up, perfume and false nails, and especially on the market-leading Bratz dolls, which tend to sport 'raunchy' clothing and make-up that some see as redolent of the sex industry. The Playboy company has been heavily criticized for apparently selling branded goods such as stationery and clothing adorned with its 'bunny' logo in the children's market. Meanwhile, newspaper headlines make much of (perhaps apocryphal) examples such as the supermarket chain that allegedly sold a pole-dancing kit in its 'Toys and Games' section, schools banning girls from wearing thongs or 'Miss Sexy' trousers, and girls wearing 'shag bands' on their wrists to signal their availability for particular sexual acts.[1]

In the last few years alone, there have been several popular books for parents addressing the sexualization of girls, mostly published in the United States (e.g. Durham, 2009; Lamb and Brown, 2006; Levin and Kilbourne, 2008; Reist, 2009), and the topic is explored by several of the campaigners discussed in chapter 1 (e.g. Mayo and Nairn, 2009; Quart, 2003). This issue has also been addressed at the level of public policy. The Australian government recently conducted a national inquiry on the sexualization of children, seemingly provoked by a controversial report entitled *Corporate Paedophilia* produced by the Australia Institute, an independent policy 'think tank' (Rush and La Nauze, 2006; and Australian Senate, 2007). In Britain, the Home Office has also commissioned and published a report in this area, undertaken by the celebrity psychologist Dr Linda Papadopoulos (Home Office, 2010); while the then Prime Minister Gordon Brown supported a campaign called 'Let Girls be Girls', launched in January 2010 by the influential parenting website mumsnet, which aims to prevent retailers from selling products that 'prematurely sexualize' children. The Conservative leader and now Prime Minister David Cameron has also remarked on the 'creepy sexualisation' of children in advertising and 'unsuitable' pop music – although he has been quite frank about his own daughter's resistance to his attempts to censor her preferences.[2] Meanwhile, in the United States, the American Psychological Association has established a Task Force on the Sexualization of Girls, whose report offers a comprehensive review of the psychological literature (American Psychological Association, 2007). While most of this concern focuses specifically on girls, some of it (as in the case of the *Corporate Paedophilia* report) extends to boys as well.

A history of concern

To some extent, these developments can be seen as a consequence of the blurring of age distinctions – the phenomenon of 'age compression' or 'kids getting older younger' that has recently become a familiar trope among marketers (see chapter 5). Yet the sexualization of children is by no means a new issue. Writers such as James Kincaid (1992, 1998) and Anne Higonnet (1998) have traced a long history of children and young people being represented as objects for erotic contemplation (and commodification) by adults. Higonnet analyses eroticized images of children in Romantic painting, book illustrations of the Victorian era, art photography and early advertising, as well as more contemporary material, while Kincaid (1998) traces a similar history in literature and film, from *Huckleberry Finn* and Lewis Carroll, through *Heidi* and Shirley Temple films, to contemporary Hollywood productions such as *Home Alone*. It is perhaps worth recalling here that the age of consent for heterosexual sex in the UK was only raised from 12 to 16 in the late nineteenth century; and that child prostitutes, some as young as 8 or 9, were common in mid-nineteenth-century London (Kehily and Montgomery, 2002). While the *public visibility* of the issue, and the terms in which it is defined, may have changed, sexualized representations of children cannot be seen merely as a consequence of contemporary consumerism.

Anxieties around this issue also have a long history. Danielle Egan and Gail Hawkes (2007, 2010; Hawkes and Egan, 2008) have traced the history of concerns about childhood sexualization, for example in campaigns around 'child purity' in the late nineteenth century, the 'social hygiene' movement of the early twentieth century and the child-rearing manuals of the 1930s and 1940s. As they suggest, these concerns were often reinforced by the medicalization of childhood sexuality: the authority and expertise of developmental psychologists, physicians and sexologists were drawn upon to justify the close supervision and regulation of children's sexual instincts. Egan and Hawkes argue that such concerns reflect a strange ambivalence about childhood sexuality: it is both denied (because children are deemed to be innocent) and yet seen as a potentially unstoppable force once it is 'released' by external corrupting influences.

Dan Cook and Susan Kaiser (2004) point to similar kinds of concerns emerging in popular debates in the 1960s and 1970s. As they suggest, this was in part a response to the creation of new age-defined categories such as the 'teenager' and the 'subteen' in the post-war clothing market. The rapid increase in numbers among this age group as a result of the so-called 'baby boom' precipitated some confusion among marketers about how it should be targeted; and particular products or aspects of marketing – from the Barbie doll through to Calvin Klein's notorious campaign featuring the teenage Brooke Shields ('nothing comes between me and my Calvins') – attracted widespread public criticism for their implicit or explicit sexual connotations.[3] As Cook and Kaiser suggest, marketing to the 'tween' market is also characterized by considerable ambiguity, especially in relation to sexuality: marketers have to walk a difficult line between showing girls as 'attractive' and presenting them as 'sexy' (see also Walkerdine, 1997).

Egan and Hawkes (2008) argue that there are considerable continuities between these historical campaigns and contemporary concerns – for example, those emerging around the Australia Institute report. 'Sexualisation', they suggest, is often seen here in highly deterministic, monolithic terms; and when it comes to the influence of media and marketing, this is regarded as a 'hypodermic' process, in which children are passive victims rather than active meaning-makers. They argue that the consequence of such arguments is to deny the sexual agency of girls in particular: girls' sexuality (or sexual expression) is equated with sexualization, and cannot be imagined outside the context of exploitative commercial messages. According to these authors, there is also a strong class dimension here: it is the sexuality of *working-class* girls that is seen as particularly problematic and in need of discipline and control.

It is important to note here that such changes are not merely cultural in nature, or indeed simply constructed by the market. The age of physical and sexual maturity has fallen significantly over the past century. The age of menarche (onset of menstruation) in the United States and Europe dropped by around 2.5 years in the first part of the twentieth century, although this seems to have levelled off in recent decades (Eveleth, 1986). However, the onset of puberty (for example, as indicated in breast development and the growth of pubic hair) appears to be occurring ever earlier – although this also varies according to body mass and ethnicity (Aksglaede et al., 2008; Kaplowitz et al., 2001). Around one-third of 7-year-old girls are now showing pubertal characteristics – a phenomenon that may itself cast some light both on the creation of the 'tween' market and on the resurgence of debates about sexualization.

A problem area

There are two significant problems in addressing this area. The first is that it seems to bring together some rather disparate issues. The broad concern about sexualization seems to combine anxieties about the effects on children (the apparent corruption of childhood innocence) with fears about the effects on adults (most spectacularly in the case of paedophilia and child abuse). Exposing children to sexual material is believed by some to create a premature or inappropriate interest in sex, and also to promote a range of unsafe sexual practices. The issue of body image overlaps with this: children (particularly girls) are seen to be under pressure to have slender, 'sexy' bodies, invoking concerns about gender stereotyping as well as more specific fears about threats to physical and mental health (as in the case of eating disorders). Some of these concerns relate to physical health and behaviour, some to attitudes, and some to moral values; some are quite specific, while others are much more generalized; some potentially apply to everyone, while others relate to events or conditions that may be relatively rare. While it would seem important to separate out these issues, doing so is by no means straightforward.

The second major difficulty here is the intense emotions that these issues seem to provoke. As Stevi Jackson (1982) and others note, sexuality is a key dimension of the distinction between childhood and adulthood: despite Freud's 'discovery' of infantile sexuality, the image of the sexual (or 'sexualized') child fundamentally threatens our sense of what children should be. Even more disturbingly, it raises the spectre of adults' own unconscious desire for children's bodies: it transgresses the boundaries that define how adults are supposed to look at children. James Kincaid's work on the Victorian sexualization of children (Kincaid, 1992) is particularly troubling in this respect: it implies that the post-Romantic construction of the innocent child is itself a manifestation of an unspoken (and unspeakable) adult desire. At the same time, there are questions here about how 'sex' itself is defined: what adults perceive as sexual may not be perceived as such (or in the same way) by children. As the work of authors such as Michel Foucault (e.g. 1978) and Jeffrey Weeks (e.g. 1981) has indicated, the domain of the sexual is socially, culturally and historically defined in many different ways – to the extent where any appeal to 'natural' or 'healthy' sexuality must be seen as highly problematic.

Campaigners' concerns

As with obesity and the broader arguments about children and consumption, it is important to trace the ways in which the 'problem' of sexualization is socially defined and constructed. Here again, we can identify key claims-makers or 'moral entrepreneurs' who are active in framing the issue and sustaining its public visibility (see chapter 1). In the process, we can also trace the mobilization of assumptions and discourses about childhood itself, and the ways in which alternative interpretations of the phenomenon are marginalized.

The book *So Sexy So Soon: The New Sexualised Childhood and What Parents Can Do to Protect Their Kids* (Levin and Kilbourne, 2008) provides a useful index of some of the more intense concerns that appear to be at stake here. According to these authors, children's exposure to media and commercial marketing results in their being prematurely induced into inappropriate forms of sexual behaviour. The concern here relates partly to children's viewing of media material designed for an older audience (such as music videos and pornography), and partly to material explicitly targeting them (such as teen/tween magazines, clothing and toys). The primary focus here is on girls, who are seen to be preoccupied with the need to appear sexually attractive at an ever-younger age, although such material is also believed to affect boys' attitudes towards girls, and increasingly boys' own self-image. The authors argue that the sexualization of childhood has a range of damaging consequences for children's mental and physical health – leading to depression and suicide, eating disorders and child abuse – as well as for family relationships.

The account that is offered here is resolutely one-dimensional. The authors' terminology represents children as passive victims of attack by an all-powerful media and consumer culture: children are seen to be assaulted, bombarded, victimized and deeply harmed; while the material they are exposed to is described as obscene, destructive and evil. Children are 'remotely controlled' by media, 'programmed like robots'. Media and marketing are accused of trivializing and objectifying sex, imposing rigid and unchanging gender stereotypes, promoting 'casual' sex and neglecting the 'healthy', 'human' aspects of relationships: indeed, according to these authors, there is 'never any emphasis on relationships or intimacy' in media representations. These criticisms are by no means confined to 'adult' media: even relatively tame material such as Disney's *High School Musical* is seen as equally to blame. Drawing on deficit models of child development, the authors represent children as vulnerable, unsophisticated, and as passively 'shaped' by this relentless 'onslaught' of inappropriate messages. Parents appear equally powerless: their authority is comprehensively undermined by the media's appeal to premature adolescent rebellion and their incitement of 'pester power'.

The notion of 'sexualization' is defined in various ways here. On one level, the term seems to imply that children are naturally non-sexual, but that they have been somehow *made* sexual through their exposure to media and marketing: sexuality is being inappropriately imposed upon them, rather than chosen by them. Sexualization is also seen to entail 'objectification', or 'the reduction of people to objects': objectification apparently equates a person's value, or their attractiveness, with their degree of sexual appeal. Such 'sexualized' or 'objectifying' representations are compared with those that are deemed to be 'healthy' – although healthy sexuality is defined in rather vague terms, as somehow more 'holistic' or more 'human'.

There are several difficulties here. These authors fail to provide any examples that would help to explain what a sexual *but not sexualized* representation would be like, and, by default, the two concepts seem to become conflated – any representation that may be seen (by adults) to carry sexual connotations is automatically defined as 'sexualizing'. Further, one could argue that all visual representations necessarily 'objectify'; and some would even suggest that sexual desire is bound to entail some dimension of 'objectification' – although since the characteristics of objectification are not clear, it is genuinely hard to know. There are obviously considerable variations in what people find sexually arousing – or indeed what they define as 'sexual' in the first place, let alone what they perceive as objectifying, or as 'human'. This is not merely a matter of academic sophistry. If there is a suggestion that either the government or parents should intervene to proscribe certain kinds of material, then it is important to have very clear criteria for doing so. In the case of pornography, and indeed in the area of film classification, these criteria already exist; but when such criteria involve nebulous and ambiguous concepts like these, it is genuinely difficult to see how they might be implemented.

Similar problems are apparent in other popular texts on sexualization. Meenakshi Durham's *The Lolita Effect* (2009) focuses on a series of 'myths' that are apparently imposed on girls by the commercial media. Girls are encouraged to believe that they should 'flaunt' their sexuality, that they should conform to narrowly defined and unrealistic body shapes, and that violence and sex work are somehow 'sexy'. In the process, their 'natural', 'normal', 'healthy' sexuality is being systematically denied, narrowed and distorted. Like Levin and Kilbourne, Durham represents the media as an irresistible force, bombarding, manipulating and exploiting girls and women; and here again, there is an apparently seamless continuum linking Miley Cyrus or *The Lion King* with child pornography and sex trafficking. Even so, there are some contradictions in this apparently monolithic account. Durham's academic background is in Media Studies, and she is keen to acknowledge that girls are discriminating and critical users of media – although she ultimately falls back on simplistic models of media effects, in which girls are seen as simply duped by these 'compelling role models'. While attempting to maintain a 'sex positive' stance, and to avoid 'victim feminism', she also seeks to prescribe the acceptable forms of 'healthy' sexuality, which it seems can only be experienced somewhere *outside* the world of consumer culture.

Although such concerns are apparent in other cultural contexts, it is important to recognize that they do take different forms. The debate in the United States in particular is dominated by the religious Right – although liberal feminist authors such as Levin and Kilbourne (2008) are keen to exempt themselves from charges of 'prudishness', asserting that their concerns are essentially to do with children's 'emotional health' rather than with morality. By contrast, opinion surveys in the UK (such as those conducted by the Broadcasting Standards Council: see Bragg and Buckingham, 2002) tend to suggest that British adults are increasingly permissive in their responses to sexual content, at least on television. It is hard to imagine that an incident like Janet Jackson's infamous 'wardrobe malfunction' during the 2004 Superbowl would have attracted anything like the attention in the UK that it did in the US. However, it is also worth noting that teenage pregnancy in the US is much more prevalent than in the UK. Contraceptive use is lower in the US than in Europe, while rates of sexually transmitted diseases are significantly higher. Meanwhile (and not coincidentally), sex education programmes have until recently been required to follow an 'abstinence-based' approach (Levine, 2002). If we compare the different ways in which these issues are addressed in the broader European and global context, it becomes clear that the concern about 'sexualization' is itself quite culturally specific.[4]

Feminist perspectives

As with campaigns against pornography, the public debate about sexualization often seems to involve a somewhat awkward alliance here between what might loosely be termed advocates of conservative morality (on the one hand) and feminist critics (on the other). However, it is important to note that there is no singular 'feminist' position on this issue.

For some feminists, the increasing sexualization of girls and young women is clearly seen as part of an anti-feminist 'backlash'. It represents a response on the part of male-dominated media and cultural industries to the growing power and assertiveness of women, which are evident in a whole range of domains from politics and business to education (Levy, 2006). Encouraging girls to take an unnecessary or excessive interest in their physical appearance, and to judge themselves primarily in terms of their attractiveness to men, is interpreted as a means of reasserting male oppression. For popular authors such as Naomi Wolf (1990), the 'myth' or 'cult' of physical beauty promoted through the media, advertising and fashion industries is seen to induce shame, guilt, confusion and neurosis: girls and women are perceived here very much as passive victims of a form of psychological and ideological manipulation.

However, other feminists argue that this approach denies women's agency and autonomy, presenting them merely as dupes of male power; and they also criticize such arguments for colluding with forms of conservative morality or 'decency' that have typically sought to constrain women's expressions of their independent sexuality. Linda Duits and Liesbet van Zoonen (2006) argue that older feminists' criticisms of the sexualization of girls' fashion are hypocritical in seeking to distinguish between the 'good' political style of 1960s miniskirts and the 'bad' consumerist style of modern girls' fashion. They argue that girls themselves do not necessarily equate nudity (or the revelation of flesh through garments like thongs and 'crop-tops') with sexuality; and that girls who wear such apparently 'sexualized' or 'porno-chic' clothing are doing so as an expression of their own free choice and autonomy, and not as the result of false consciousness (see also Duits and van Zoonen, 2007).

A third – equally 'feminist' – position can be found in Ros Gill's (2007) response to these arguments. Gill argues that this celebration of girls' choice and autonomy represents a dangerous form of 'post-feminism' that is complicit with neo-liberal individualism: far from representing free choice, such practices (along with other aspects of contemporary young women's 'beauty regimes' such as waxing, bleaching and cosmetic surgery) are essentially a consequence of consumerism (see also Gill, 2008). In many respects, this debate replays broader discussions within feminism about the political significance of so-called 'girl power' – the commercial marketing of a particular version of assertive, apparently 'sexualized' femininity popularized in the late 1990s by the Spice Girls, and evident across a wide range of cultural phenomena (see Harris, 2004b).

These different positions also reflect different interpretations of the broader 'sexualization' of contemporary culture that are apparent in recent social theory (Attwood, 2007). There has been a considerable amount of discussion here of the 'mainstreaming', or increasingly widespread circulation and appropriation, of sexual imagery within popular culture and public discourse. Several commentators have pointed to the growing visibility and accessibility of sexual representations, products and services, and to the increasing diversity and self-reflexivity of this phenomenon. Some authors regard this as a 'democratisation of desire', a progressive means through which more diverse sexual identities can be represented (McNair, 2002; Weeks, 2007). However, others (such as Gill, 2008) suggest that it is merely a renewed form of male oppression, in which women's apparent 'empowerment' has been commodified, and which reinforces the need for women to police their own physical appearance. Attwood (2007) argues that there are elements of truth in both accounts: while she challenges the feminist tendency to play down social change – and hence to see new developments as merely a continuation of the 'same old story' of male oppression – she is also wary of the easy celebration of a new sexual democracy. As this implies, the apparent 'sexualization' of children needs to be seen in the light of broader social and historical changes, not just in the social position of children or in the general visibility of sexuality within culture, but also in the nature of identity or individuality in 'late modern' societies (see, for example, Giddens (1992) and N. Rose (1999)).

Parents' views

While popular authors such as Levin and Kilbourne (2008) and Durham (2009) often purport to speak on behalf of parents, it is important to beware of assuming that they are necessarily representative of parents in general. Together with colleagues, I conducted a qualitative study of this issue, which included a series of deliberative focus groups with parents in Scotland (Bragg and Buckingham, forthcoming). In general, it appeared that 'sexualized' products were not necessarily a major problem for the parents in our study, as compared with other matters. Some argued that 'little has changed', that children have always wanted to 'grow up too soon' and to experiment with adult identities – although they felt that there was new and growing pressure from commercialization. Nevertheless, parents also recognized children's expertise in the codes of contemporary consumer culture – and even that their own comparative incompetence here could undermine the authority of their views.

Most parents talked about childhood in terms of 'innocence', but interpretations of this varied. Some saw experimenting with make-up, even imitating 'sexy' dance styles (and similar behaviour) as innocuous, natural, fun and devoid of adult sexual connotations. For others, innocence meant play untroubled by concerns about the adult world, which made the same activities distasteful. Parents generally saw children as passing through 'natural' stages of development towards adulthood, which required them gradually to take on increasing responsibilities. In addition, most held broadly 'democratic' ideals of child rearing, recognizing children's rights to make their own decisions, develop their individuality and express themselves. Many parents argued that disagreements over issues such as make-up or clothes did not merit jeopardizing or damaging their relationship with their children. They were seen not only as comparatively trivial, but also as a predictable developmental stage, involving rebellion and experimentation. As a result, many parents accepted that by secondary school, or around the age of 12 or 13, children should if they wished have the final say on clothes and items of personal care.

In this study, the debate about sexualized goods raised different concerns in relation to daughters as compared with sons. Parents were concerned about their daughters' psychological wellbeing, although none of them felt their *own* daughters were becoming 'too sexual too soon' and they denied that products alone could sexualize them. However, girls were thought to put themselves at risk if they appeared older than they were or dressed in sexualized ways. Boys' consumption and developing sexual identities were generally viewed in a far more relaxed way. Parents' existing strategies for dealing with sexualized products were mostly indirect and non-coercive. In general, they felt that regulation would be unlikely to be effective, not least because of the difficulty of coming to agreement about the meaning of any single item. Ultimately, they tended to conclude that it was their own responsibility to take action on sexualized products, if they so chose. However, they also revealed how difficult this was in practice, for several reasons: the availability of the products; peer pressure or general adolescent culture; children's 'nagging' and persuasive tactics; decisions made by other parents or institutions (such as schools); and economic structures and values limiting choice and shaping tastes. For these parents, the market undoubtedly did play a role in the formation of sexual identities, but it was seen to do this in complex ways, and in the context of other processes and influences. As this implies, parents' views on these matters may well be much more nuanced and ambivalent than those of the campaigners who claim to speak on their behalf.

Media effects research

To what extent does the evidence from research support campaigners' claims about the sexualization of girls? The recent high-profile reports by the Australia Institute (Rush and La Nauze, 2006) and the American Psychological Association (2007) both provide extensive reviews of the psychological literature on sexualization, and consider the role of the media (and, to a lesser extent, marketing and consumer goods) alongside other influences such as parents and peers. Yet both exemplify some of the continuing problems of mainstream media effects research in addressing such issues, which have been considered in earlier chapters. Three overarching problems can be identified here.[5]

The first relates to the analysis of *media content*. It would be hard to deny that sexual content in mainstream media has increased, and become more explicit, in recent years; and that sexual imagery has become more widely circulated within society more broadly, including in advertising and in the design and packaging of goods and services. This is also true, to a much more limited extent, of media and products targeted directly at children – and, in any case, it forms part of the broader environment in which children are currently growing up (see also Arthurs, 2004; Attwood, 2009; Bragg and Buckingham, 2002).

However, there is room for further debate about the nature of these representations and the 'messages' they convey. The Australia Institute report, for example, discusses a range of media content, including advertisements for children's clothing, sample editions of teen or tween magazines, and popular television programmes. In the case of the advertisements, the analysis suggests that children (both boys and girls) are increasingly being posed and represented in ways that used to apply to adult models – an approach the authors describe as 'grotesque'. In the case of the teen magazines, the authors seek to quantify the amount of 'sexualising material'; while in the case of television, they point to the 'high degree of sexual innuendo' in music videos and television shows like *Big Brother* and *The O.C.* Yet the report fails to differentiate between 'sexual' and 'sexualized' (or 'objectifying') representations: it would seem that any reference to sex or intimate relationships, and almost any representation of a human body or body part, is perceived by the authors as 'sexualized'. This results in some readings that can only be described as extremely partial. Even more disturbingly, the authors seem to read strongly adult connotations into images of children: as Lumby and Albury (2008) put it, they imply that 'dressing young girls in crop tops or bikinis carries the same cultural messages as dressing a mature adult woman in identical clothing'.

Likewise, most of the content analyses cited in the APA report make no distinction between 'sexual' and 'sexualized' content: most simply code all 'sexual' content. Yet the studies cited do not adopt the same criteria for defining such content: for example, one study codes 'women dancing sexually', another looks at whether women are 'suggestively dressed', while another looks at whether we see athletes' breasts or their faces. In some instances, it appears that any image of a body part (as opposed to a whole body) is an instance of 'dismembering', and hence of sexualization – a criterion that might apply to a vast range of images, including many images of men. It is also not clear how the judgement of 'sexual appeal' or 'physical attractiveness' is made, and on what basis.

There is a familiar tendency here (equivalent to that in research on media violence) to assume that the *meaning* of 'sexual' or 'sexualized' images is fixed and can be taken for granted (and hence simply quantified). It seems to be assumed, for example, that when a person is shown in a 'sexualized' manner, this is necessarily presented as a positive attribute of their character, and as something to be emulated. 'Sexualized' images are also compared with a norm of 'healthy' representation that seems indifferent to questions of genre or realism, which results in some strangely inappropriate judgements: for example, music videos are condemned for failing to show 'the concept of a whole person involved in a complex relationship with another whole person' (p. 7), while children's dolls are condemned for not displaying 'healthy', 'normal' sexuality (p. 14). There are some striking differences in these respects between the kinds of content analysis drawn upon here and the forms of *textual* analysis developed by cultural critics. Like the popular campaigners discussed above, these reports present media and marketing as a kind of ideological monolith – as containing and imposing a consistent and coherent set of 'messages', with little change or complexity. By contrast, Media Studies critics suggest that contemporary media messages about youth and sexuality are much more diverse, and often contradictory (e.g. Arthurs, 2004; G. Davis and Dickinson, 2004; Kaveney, 2006).

Evidence about media content cannot in itself be taken as evidence of its effects on consumers; and this takes us to the second key problem here. It is obviously likely that children will be influenced by dominant ideas about physical attractiveness and 'sexiness' (although these are not necessarily seen as the same thing). Yet in fact almost all of the research on the *impact* of this material cited in the reports relates to adults (particularly university students) rather than children. There is very little evidence here that would enable us to assess how far adults' perceptions of what is sexual are shared by children – or indeed how children themselves interpret and deal with what they see and consume, and how they use this in their everyday lives.

The APA report (2007) cites a range of evidence in support of its conclusion that sexualized images of women have negative consequences, in terms of girls' cognitive functioning and educational achievement, their physical and mental health (for example anxiety, shame, self-disgust, eating disorders, low self-esteem and depression), their attitudes and beliefs, and their ability to develop 'healthy' sexuality. The report does not offer any critique of the many studies it cites, beyond drawing attention to apparent gaps in the field. Rather, it takes them at face value, as 'evidence' that can simply be amassed and then weighed up. Needless to say perhaps, the well-known methodological criticisms that have been raised in relation to media effects research (as discussed in chapter 3) are ignored. The reliance on laboratory experiments, which focus exclusively on short-term effects, would seem particularly inappropriate in relation to an apparently long-term, pervasive phenomenon like sexualization. Here again, the discussion of questionnaire surveys repeatedly presents evidence of correlations or associations (for example, between exposure to specific types of media and aspects of physical or mental health) as though they represented causal relationships.

Furthermore, many of the studies cited are not in fact explicitly concerned with 'sexualization' at all: they cover a broad range of issues from body image and eating disorders, self-esteem and self-concept to sexual harassment, as well as beliefs about sexuality. Depending on how it is defined, sexualization might be seen to play a part in these areas, but it is not synonymous with them: for example, body dissatisfaction or eating disorders may have multiple causes which may be nothing to do with sexuality. 'Sexualization' is essentially a *post hoc* construct, which is retrospectively applied to the studies cited; nor is it at all clear that the studies cited would share the APA's definition of sexualization.

This takes us on to the third major problem here, which is the basic *definition* (or lack of definition) of sexualization itself. According to the APA report, sexualization can be manifested through any one of four key characteristics. It occurs when: 'a person's value comes only from his or her sexual appeal or behaviour, to the exclusion of other characteristics'; 'a person is held to a standard that equates physical attractiveness (narrowly defined) with being sexy'; 'a person is sexually objectified — that is, made into a thing for others' sexual use, rather than seen as a person with the capacity for independent action and decision making'; and/or 'when sexuality is inappropriately imposed upon a person'.

This definition is both highly inclusive and very imprecise. On this basis, it would be possible to accuse almost any text featuring a physical image of a person as 'sexualizing': anything from hardcore pornography through to shampoo advertisements would have to be included (and in fact, this is the approach the report adopts). One could argue that very few advertising or fashion images (for example) ever depict people as having 'the capacity for independent action and decision making' – the people in such images are rarely 'characterized' in this way (any more than they are, for example, in paintings). Here again, the definition provides no way of distinguishing between material that is 'sexual' (that is, concerned with sexual matters, or sexually explicit) and material that is 'sexualized'. It is not clear what a *non-sexualized* image of a human body (or even parts of a human body) would be like. Nor is it clear what terms like 'narrowly defined' or – crucially, in respect of children – 'inappropriate' actually mean, or how these things might be identified. There is an assumption here that readers of the report will share a view about what is and is not 'sexual', and what is or is not 'appropriate', as well as what is deemed to be 'healthy'. While purporting to present objective scientific evidence, the report implicitly adopts a prescriptive view of such matters that it fails adequately to define or to justify.

These problems are replicated in the more recent UK government report (Home Office, 2010). Like the APA report, it asserts that there is consensus among researchers on this issue – a claim that is only possible on the basis of a highly selective and uncritical presentation of the evidence. Perhaps the most problematic aspect of this report, however, is its implicit connection between the sexualization of girls and violence against women – an argument that, with no substantial supporting evidence, comes very close to a 'blame the victim' logic.

Children's perspectives

As with other controversies about media effects, one general characteristic of this debate is that children's voices are almost entirely absent. Popular authors such as Levin and Kilbourne (2008) tend to privilege the views of 'concerned' parents, who may or may not be representative of parents at large, while the psychological research tends to focus on easily accessible groups of college students (indeed, the effects of the media on white, middle-class students following communication courses at mid-Western American universities must surely be one of the most closely scrutinized of all aspects of contemporary life). This absence is particularly crucial here, since (as I have suggested) what adults perceive to be 'sexual' (or 'sexualized') may not be perceived in the same way by children.

By contrast, my earlier research, conducted with Sara Bragg (Buckingham and Bragg, 2004) was based on extensive interviews with children aged 9–17 about their responses to representations of love, sex and relationships in television, film and print media, as well as a large-scale survey. We found that young people did quite frequently encounter sexual material in the media, although relatively little of this could be considered 'explicit'. This material was also quite diverse in terms of the 'messages' it was seen to contain: while sex was sometimes represented as pleasurable and desirable, it was also often surrounded by moral warnings about the dangers it could entail. These young people certainly did not perceive the media to be pressurizing them into adopting a merely 'recreational' attitude to sex.

In general, our respondents valued the media's role as a source of information about sex and relationships, sometimes rating them more highly than parents or (particularly) teachers: they found it less embarrassing to find out about such matters in this way, and perceived media such as teenage magazines and soap operas as being more attuned to their needs. However, this is not to say that they necessarily trusted what they found: on the contrary, they made complex judgements about the relationships between media representations and reality, engaged with the moral dilemmas of stories and characters they encountered, and were sometimes extremely critical of what they saw. At the same time, the younger children did not necessarily always understand sexual references or 'innuendoes', and often ignored or misinterpreted them: they were far from being the sexual sophisticates imagined by some conservative critics. We also found that the influence of the media depended very much on the settings in which they were used, particularly in the context of family life: parents in particular were powerful models of adult sexual identity. While this research does confirm that children learn about sexual matters from the media, it suggests that this is very far from the straightforward or inexorable process that is implied by the notion of 'sexualization'.

Similar findings emerge from other qualitative studies based on interviews or ethnographic fieldwork with children and young people. The work of Brown et al. (1993), Steele (1999) and their colleagues in the United States, Kehily's (1999) UK-based research on teenage girls' readings of magazines, and the more recent study in New Zealand by Vares and Jackson (2010) all suggest that children are far from being duped by the media into a passive acceptance of stereotyped or indeed 'sexualized' gender roles. While they can see the media as providing valuable 'resources' for learning about sex and relationships, they often read such material critically, comparing it with their own lived experience and their observation of peers and adults around them, and questioning romantic fantasies and idealized body images. Explicitly sexual material is often rejected as excessive or disgusting. While some appear fascinated by media coverage, they are keen to debate whether it can be seen as accurate or trustworthy. They also have their own complex notions about what is appropriate or 'decent', both for children of their own age, and for those who are younger; and their judgements here can be just as moralistic as those of adults who fear for their welfare (see also Kelley et al., 1999).

This research has not looked at other aspects of marketing and consumer culture. However, a few recent studies have offered some interesting insights into how girls understand and debate the wearing of apparently 'sexualized' clothing. Viveka Torell (2004) studied letters written to a Swedish young people's magazine on this issue, and found a considerable degree of ambivalence. On the one hand, girls argued that they have the right to wear such clothes, and that doing so made them feel good; but there was also considerable disagreement among them about the age at which this was appropriate. Interestingly, similar arguments were rehearsed here in relation to the current fashion for boys to wear low-slung trousers that reveal their underpants: while some saw this as excitingly rebellious, others dismissed it as merely disgusting. In addressing the same topic, Mari Rysst (2010) found in her ethnographic fieldwork in Norway that girls operated a complex and multifaceted system for classifying clothing, which reflected different values associated with both gender and social class. Significantly, clothes that many adults see as 'sexualized' were not seen as such by children, but rather as merely 'cool' and fashionable. As in our earlier research, there was a sense here in which some children were actively refusing adult perceptions of such clothes as 'sexy' (see also Buckingham and Bragg, 2005). In the UK, Jane Pilcher (2010) encountered a similar ambivalence among 6- to 11-year-old girls: while some enjoyed dressing up in fashionable clothing, and saw it as a way of 'ageing up' towards feminine adulthood (albeit only in restricted domestic contexts, and after discussions with parents), they also displayed some anxiety and disapproval of 'revealing' clothing. Even here, however, it was far from clear that the girls recognized the specifically sexual implications of such clothing, or showed a strong sense of to whom their showing of the body might be directed: the issue was formulated more as a matter of 'modesty' than of sexual provocation.

In another relevant study, Rebekah Willett (2008) investigated girls' uses of online 'doll-maker' sites as a means of exploring their perceptions of body image and sexual politics. The early teenage girls in her study were very self-consciously critical about these issues, and presented themselves as entirely able to resist the 'tyranny of slenderness' – although they also differentiated themselves from invisible 'others' whom they believed to be more at risk of negative media influences. While Willett's account rejects the view that girls are simply dupes of consumer culture, she also challenges the emphasis on 'compulsory individuality' that she sees as characteristic of contemporary neo-liberal discourses. The girls ultimately saw the maintenance of a slender, healthy body as an individual responsibility, a matter of self-surveillance and self-discipline (cf. Harris, 2004a). In this context, Willett argues that, far from being free to 'express themselves', the forms of young people's expression are in fact being regulated in ever more subtle ways.

In another part of our Scottish study (Buckingham et al., 2010), we conducted a series of classroom activities and focus groups with young people in their early teens in order to explore their perceptions of potentially 'sexualized' products. Here again, these young people rejected the idea that they were passive victims of the marketing of such goods; and this claim was to a large extent supported both by their extensive knowledge of marketing techniques and by the examples they provided of their active choices and careful judgements about products. They indicated that their knowledge about how to 'read' products such as clothing and accessories developed as they grew older, and was informed by peer culture as they entered wider social settings (such as high school). They were also aware of the risks of appearing older through the use of sexualized products and generally having personal appearances misread. The perceived risks ranged from paedophilia to general risks about reputation and misjudgements – risks that related far more to girls than to boys.

These young people recognized that they were influenced to some degree by fashion trends and by their peers; and yet, somewhat contradictorily, they argued that their purchases were also part of their expression of individuality. Their choices in relation to 'sexualized' goods reflected peer group norms to do with inclusion and exclusion, and with feelings of comfort and confidence. These norms involved complicated value systems relating to taste, and to the perceived meanings of particular objects or products. For example, it was generally considered normative not to display too much of the body or to draw attention to oneself through hairstyles, make-up and accessories. Apparent 'failures' of taste or style were typically seen to be characteristic of *other* people, who were often referred to in derogatory terms relating to social class (such as 'chav'). (These issues will be considered more fully in chapter 9.) Here again, there were some familiar gender differences. Girls said they were inclined to scrutinize each other's appearance more closely than boys, partly as a way of defining and confirming their own taste and identity. Boys also said they felt pressure to have a particular body shape and to consume particular goods, although current boys' trends are largely towards loose-fitting clothing that does not accentuate the body.

These young people were keen to assert that they were competent in understanding and interpreting the sexual connotations of particular products, and in assessing this dimension relative to other concerns. They strongly rejected the idea that regulation was necessary in order to protect them, and argued that they should have the right to make their own decisions (and mistakes). However, they also expected adults to provide 'correct' guidance – and here again, they condemned parents of *other* children and teenagers who were acting irresponsibly by failing to regulate their children's choices.

Of course, it is vital not to take children's testimony at face value. As Gill (2007) points out, there is a danger here of presenting their relationships with media and consumer culture simply as a matter of them exercising 'free choice'. Yet, on the other hand, as Duits and van Zoonen (2007) argue, we should be careful not to deny children's agency in these matters. The research I have cited here is by no means naïve about this: on the contrary, it typically presents children's discussions of media and consumer culture as an arena for complex forms of 'identity work'. It also helps to move beyond simplistic models of media effects, suggesting that the media do not have an autonomous power either to corrupt children or, indeed, to 'liberate' them.

Conclusion

It is undoubtedly the case that sexual imagery has become more widely available within the culture as a whole, including in material that is targeted at, or frequently consumed by, children. However, the evidence about the *effects* of this – whether positive or negative – is limited and inconclusive. Media effects research, of the kind that is frequently cited by campaigners in this area, seems particularly ill equipped to address the complexity of the issues at stake. These limitations are partly to do with the scope of the research, and the methods that have been employed; but they are primarily to do with the lack of consistency and clarity about the meaning of 'sexualization' itself. Much of the research rests on moral assumptions – for example about 'healthy' sexuality, about 'decency' or about material that is 'inappropriate' for children – that are not adequately explained or justified.

By contrast, the studies I have discussed in the later sections of this chapter adopt a different approach. They confirm that the media and marketing do play a key role in children's developing understanding of sexuality, and that this is generally more problematic for girls than for boys. However, they suggest that this role can be positive as well as negative. If the media exert 'pressure' on children, this is not simply about imposing inappropriate values: rather, the problem is that children have to find their own way through a diverse range of potentially contradictory or inconsistent messages, deriving both from the media and from other sources (Buckingham and Bragg, 2005). This would imply that they need opportunities to engage with these issues in a context that is not unduly dominated by moral judgements or by the perspectives of adults. To this extent, the sensationalizing terms in which the debate about sexualization tends to be conducted might be seen as positively counter-productive for children themselves.

8

Rethinking 'pester power'
· Children, parents and consumption

Parents obviously play a central role in children's engagements with consumer culture. Especially for younger children, it is parents (along with grandparents and other family members) who provide the economic resources for the large majority of children's purchasing and consumption. Most of children's spending is in fact *parents'* spending: it is parents who pay, even if it is children who consume or use what they buy. Much of this does not involve choice on the part of children, or even consultation with them. Babies are 'consumers' of commercial goods well before they can speak; and indeed parents consume on behalf of children when preparing for their birth. Even when it comes to older children, most of their purchasing is actually made possible by gifts from adults. Parents still exert much more influence on what children – especially young children – buy and consume than vice versa.

As we have seen, parents feature in some paradoxical ways in the popular debate about children's consumption. Many of the campaigning publications are addressed explicitly to parents, and call on them to take up arms against the negative consequences of consumer culture (see chapter 1). While children are typically seen here as vulnerable and incompetent, parents too are represented as effectively powerless against the onslaught of commercial forces – although they are also frequently blamed for their failure to resist them. 'Permissive' parents are seen to be particularly at fault for surrendering to their children's apparently uncontrollable consumer desires. 'Responsible' parents, meanwhile, are engaged in a constant struggle to contain and control their children's exposure to marketing and commercial values.

Marketers are also very much aware of the influence of parents on children's consumer behaviour. Marketing texts typically categorize the range of parenting styles and provide recommendations on how they can be addressed: Sutherland and Thompson (2001), for example, distinguish between 'Indulgers', 'Conflicted', 'Kids' Pals' and 'Bare Necessities', and suggest likely strategies in each case (see also Siegel et al., 2001). In general, marketers regard the more egalitarian approach of contemporary parenting as a significant marketing opportunity – although when campaigners challenge what they see as the exploitation of children, marketers are quick to respond by saying that it is down to parents to take charge and to control their children's consumption (Schor, 2004).

In previous chapters, I have argued that children's consumption should not be seen in individualistic terms. On the contrary, it is unavoidably embedded in networks of social relationships (cf. Chin, 2001; Cook, 2008). Parents are key actors in these networks, performing a variety of roles as providers, enablers, regulators, gatekeepers, teachers, and so on. From the moment of a child's conception, parents are consumers on behalf of children; but the child can also act as a vehicle or a focus for parents' own consumer desires. Historically, this relationship has been characterized by a considerable degree of ambivalence: children's consumption acts as a repository for a whole range of parents' fears and fantasies, as well as for changing ideas about what makes 'good parenting' (see chapter 4). This ambivalence is certainly apparent in parents' and children's negotiations over key areas such as food and clothing, considered in the previous two chapters; and in the area of education, which will be addressed in chapter 11.

This chapter addresses the role of consumption in parent/child relationships in three main ways. Firstly, I argue that we need to understand this phenomenon in the context of broader historical changes in family life – in family structures, in the ways in which families manage time and space in the home, and in ideologies of parenting. All of these have contributed to a general shift in the power relationships of contemporary families, which have significant implications in terms of consumption. Following from this, I argue secondly that this process is more complex than a simple power struggle between two (or three) unequal contenders: rather, the negotiations that surround children's consumption are much more complex than is suggested by popular notions such as 'pester power'. Finally, I argue that parents themselves are also inevitably invested in consumer culture. Their relationships with their children (their feelings of love and care, as well as their anxieties, hopes and aspirations) are inextricably tied up with consumer desires. However, I also suggest that social class is a key issue here, and that these relationships operate in increasingly fraught ways in a context of growing social inequality. In focusing on relationships between parents and children, this chapter is principally concerned with younger children, while the next chapter, which takes a similar approach to the peer group, focuses rather more on older children in the pre-teen and teen age groups.

The family in crisis?

As we saw in chapter 1, some popular commentators have suggested that the contemporary family is 'in crisis' – although such claims themselves also have a long history. Parenting has become a significant focus for public debate and for policy interventions: there is a rising sense of anxiety about the failure of modern parents, and growing calls for increased surveillance. Critics frequently point to what they perceive as a widespread collapse of parental discipline, and the tendency for parents to prioritize the demands of work over those of 'family time', while others are keen to condemn what they regard as an unduly protective, even 'paranoid', approach to child rearing (e.g. Furedi, 2008; O. James, 2010; S. Palmer, 2006). It is partly because of this apparent crisis or failure on the part of parents that commercial forces are seen to be having an increasingly powerful role in childhood.

However, the reality is more complex and more ambivalent. Melodramatic claims about the demise of traditional family life are, to say the least, overstated. While there have certainly been significant changes here (which one might see as both positive and negative), nostalgia for an imagined 'Golden Age' of family harmony and togetherness is largely misplaced. In the following sections, I outline some of the broader social changes that have characterized family life over the past few decades. My account here relates specifically to the UK, although readers from other countries will probably recognize points of comparison (there have certainly been similar changes in the US, for example: see Pugh, 2009). Much of the information here is drawn from social statistics, which permit some kind of systematic comparison over a fifty-year period.[1]

In contemporary Britain, the structure and composition of families are certainly changing, although not as radically or as rapidly as some commentators suggest. Over the past fifty years, family structures have in general become 'longer and thinner': most families contain fewer dependent children (as birth-rates have fallen), but children tend to remain in the family home for a longer period. Although alternative forms of family organization have become more common, over three-quarters of children still live in a nuclear family unit, with two parents (including step-parents). Household sizes have generally fallen, with a particular decline in large households – although the latter are more common among some ethnic groups. Women are having children later in life, and this is correlated with the rise in employment opportunities for women. Increasing numbers of children are born outside of marriage (over 40 per cent). Marriage rates have steadily declined since the 1970s; and divorce rates have increased overall, but are currently in decline. The number of lone parent families has increased significantly (trebling between 1971 and 2007), and an increasing number of children (currently around one in ten) live with step-parents. Children are now likely to remain in the parental home for longer than in the past, not least because of rising costs of accommodation: the majority do not leave home permanently until they are well into their twenties (ESRC, 2006; Office of National Statistics, 2007).

These developments have several potential implications for families' and children's consumption. The overall reduction in family size means that correspondingly greater economic resources may be allocated to children, and children may have a greater say in family spending; but it also means that children are likely to have fewer siblings available for companionship, and may therefore be more inclined to seek solitary forms of entertainment, or to connect with friends via electronic media. Increasing financial independence for women changes the 'balance of power' within families, in ways that are bound to affect purchasing decisions. Present-day children have fewer blood relatives (such as aunts and uncles) who might buy things for them; but they are also more likely to have grandparents who may do so (and indeed, this will be correspondingly more the case where parents have divorced and remarried). At the same time, the lengthening of the family form also means that children are dependent upon parents for a greater period of time.

There is obviously considerable diversity in patterns of income and expenditure among different family structures and social groups. In general, average levels of disposable household income and wealth in the UK have risen significantly, albeit unevenly, over the past several decades: despite the reduction in household size, average inflation-adjusted household net wealth has more than doubled over the past forty years. However, economic inequality has also increased: the rich are becoming relatively richer, while a large minority of people are affected by a relative lack of material resources. Among families with children, married couples have the highest average income, followed by cohabiting couples and then lone parents: the median income of lone mothers is around one-third of that of married couples (Kiernan et al., 1998). The larger ethnic minority groups in Britain also continue to have lower levels of income than the majority White population.

Family spending has increased greatly: it is currently two and a half times higher than in 1971, taking account of inflation. Families with children spend the most, and the cost of bringing up children has risen significantly in real terms. As I have noted, one commercial estimate of the current cost of bringing up a child from birth to the age of 21 is now over £200,000 – equivalent to roughly £25 per day (Liverpool Victoria Friendly Society, 2010). There have also been substantial changes in how households allocate expenditure: more is spent on services and less on goods; and categories such as communications, leisure, holidays and 'culture' have become proportionally more important, while others such as food and clothing have become less so. While it could be concluded that 'necessities' now account for a declining proportion of household income, it could also be suggested that goods and amenities formerly seen as 'luxuries' have now come to be regarded as necessities: this might apply to commodities such as television, central heating, freezers, washing machines and cars, as well as new media such as computers and mobile phones (Rosen, 2003).

Again, the growing expenditure on leisure is unevenly distributed, with lone parent families in particular more likely to go without leisure goods or activities – such as holidays and presents at family celebrations – that more wealthy families consider as necessities. Lower-income families are generally less likely to be able to afford formal childcare arrangements. Lone parents are still most likely to be unemployed and in poverty, although this is improving somewhat as women become more involved in the labour force, albeit often in lower-paid occupations. Ethnic minorities also continue to have the lowest-paid jobs and the highest rates of unemployment, although there are major disparities between these groups.

Broadly speaking, therefore, rising levels of affluence within British society over the past fifty years have led to a growth in the scope and scale of consumption within families. However, one of the most striking aspects here is the continuing inequalities in families' wealth and income, and hence in their access to commercially provided goods and services. These inequalities of course reflect well-established inequalities based on social class, gender and ethnicity; and they are particularly apparent in relation to single-parent families, in which growing numbers of children live. Child poverty in the UK has declined somewhat over the past ten years, although it remains at one of the highest levels in the developed world: 2 million children (around one-sixth) currently live in households where no adult is employed, and there are 2.8 million UK children living in poverty. Unequal socio-economic circumstances continue to impact significantly on children's participation in education, but also on their involvement in the range of leisure and cultural activities that constitute contemporary consumer society (Ridge, 2002). The rich and the poor do not live only in different material worlds, but in different cultural and social worlds as well.

Inside the home: time and space

As we look 'inside' the family home, we can see some significant changes in how the resources of time and space are deployed. Despite concerns about work/life balance and the pressures on 'family time', the proportions of time spent in paid and unpaid work, and on leisure and recreation, have been relatively stable over time. Parents are working slightly fewer hours per week than a decade ago, although work continues to be the second most time-consuming activity after sleeping. Married women are spending more time in paid work, and mothers in particular are increasingly in paid employment: in 2006, 30 per cent of married or cohabiting mothers with children worked full-time, and 30 per cent worked part-time. Men are doing greater amounts of childcare and housework, but women still do much more, even in dual-income families. The amount of time spent on housework is decreasing, but the time spent on childcare is rising (and is reportedly much higher than in the US or elsewhere in Europe). Nevertheless, parents – particularly in dual-earning households – report experiencing 'time squeeze', with less 'free' time for personal leisure: this applies to men as well as women, although it is more acute for women.

Families are spending more time in the home, rather than less: in 2005, 70 per cent of time was spent in the home, sleeping, doing housework, watching TV or videos, listening to music and so on – although, of course, these things are not necessarily done together as a family. While this may reflect the growing domestication of leisure activities, it is also associated with increasing concerns about safety. Statistics in this area are notoriously unreliable, but it would seem that, while actual levels of crime have fallen, the fear of crime has declined less dramatically (although it has certainly declined). In reality, it is the home, rather than the street, that is the main site for crimes against children: three-quarters of those convicted for violent offences against younger children are family members. However, young people are especially at risk in public spaces as a result of their ownership of desirable products, particularly electronic goods such as mobile phones and MP3 players. This has contributed to a situation in which children's independent mobility outside the home has been steadily restricted. Fears about traffic and abduction by paedophiles mean that younger children in particular are much more likely to be driven to school, and parents tend to prefer children to be entertained in the home rather than 'playing out' in the street or in open spaces (see Valentine, 2004).

Within the family home, the allocation of space has also changed. Partly as a result of the reduction in family size, larger numbers of children now have their own bedrooms; and the widespread availability of central heating means that children are now more likely to spend time there than in shared family rooms. Children now have much more individualized access to television and other media: the large majority now have a television set in their bedrooms, and over one-third also now have internet access. Data suggest that older children in particular are now watching a good deal of television alone; but particularly in households where there is only one multi-channel set, family viewing remains common. Similar findings apply to the use of internet-linked computers and games consoles, although some other forms of new media (such as the Nintendo Wii) are being marketed precisely as means of promoting and celebrating family togetherness.

One motivation for parents to provide large amounts of media technology for their children to use in the home may well derive from the fear of crime in public spaces (Livingstone and Bovill, 1999). Yet the advent of media-rich bedroom environments also raises the spectre of new risks to children, as a result of their unsupervised access (particularly in the case of the internet): in a sense, the problem here (at least for some) is that the private space of the home has been invaded from outside by forms of media and consumerism. In this sense, one type of perceived risk has been exchanged for another. This increasingly individualized access to technology may well encourage a degree of fragmentation in family life. However, it is also the case that such technologies (most notably mobile phones and e-mail) allow connections between family members who may be physically separated – which is a major reason why parents purchase mobile phones for their children in the first place.

In some respects, then, the situation here is rather paradoxical. Hours spent on paid and unpaid work (such as housework) are slightly declining, and yet parents increasingly report experiencing 'time squeeze'. It may well be that the sensation of 'time squeeze' – or the perceived lack of 'quality time' spent with the family – arises from the growing variety and abundance of leisure activities and products available for families to consume. However, the continuing – and perhaps accelerating – symbolic 'valorization' of childhood means that there is much greater pressure on parents to spend time with their children – and indeed to be seen to enjoy doing so. In this respect, the atmosphere of rising anxiety about family life may well have had an impact on parents themselves. Parents report that they feel under much greater public scrutiny; and the appetite for parenting advice on the internet, through books and on TV is itself a growing commercial market.

In fact, the notion of 'family time' – characterized by collective leisure activities, family meals, celebrations and outings – is a relatively modern phenomenon. As we have seen (chapter 6), the family meal typically serves as one key symbolic indicator of family togetherness. While some have seen a decline in families eating meals together, the evidence here is inconclusive (Larson et al., 2006). Even so, one could argue that the notion of 'quality time' spent with children has itself been commodified – that is, seen as something that can be bought and sold. Parents may use purchases as a way of compensating for the feelings of guilt they experience as a result of not spending what they are led to regard as sufficient time with their children – even though the figures suggest that they are in fact spending more time on childcare than previous generations of parents. Parents may therefore feel a growing pressure to both produce and defend 'family time', not least by spending money on shared activities. As we shall see, they may also feel there is an urgent need to focus children's consumption on goods and activities that are seen as worthwhile or in some way improving.

Empowered children?

In different ways, all these changes have led to children becoming much more important economic actors within the family. Children have become a more significant focus of expenditure, as well as having a greater say in family decision-making. This is partly manifested in their increased access to disposable income. The giving of pocket money (or allowances) is a relatively recent practice, dating back to the mid twentieth century. It takes a variety of forms, ranging from ad hoc payments to formal weekly or monthly allowances, which are received by around two-thirds of children. In some cases, it involves no specific obligations, for example in terms of schoolwork or chores, whereas in others it can be seen as a 'wage' given in exchange for housework or work in a family business.

Estimates of the amount of pocket money children receive are rather variable, although long-term studies over the past twenty-five years suggest that it has increased in real terms, albeit only slightly (Halifax Pocket Money Survey, 2009). However, there is some evidence that ad hoc 'handouts' and gifts from parents may be increasing: some estimates suggests that the total value of these is in the region of £2.1 billion per year in the UK (Mayo and Nairn, 2009). Perhaps surprisingly, amounts of pocket money are almost totally independent of family income: pocket money thus represents a higher proportion of the income of less wealthy families, suggesting that parents in such families are more likely to go without luxuries themselves in order to provide for their children.

The giving of allowances represents an important shift from former times, when children would have been expected to hand over much of their income from employment (Cunningham, 2006). Of course, children are much less involved in paid employment today than in the nineteenth century – although, as I have noted (chapter 3), most older children engage in part-time paid work at some stage. Contrary to expectations, it appears that children from higher-income and two-parent families are more likely to work than those from lower-income and lone parent families. Such children tend to use income from work to pay for additional 'luxuries' – and, as such, much of this work is motivated by consumption. By contrast, those from more disadvantaged backgrounds often depend on such income in order to be able to participate in what most would regard as common childhood practices.

In addition to spending their own money, children are also an increasingly significant influence on parental or family purchasing decisions. While marketers have been aware of this phenomenon for many years (Jacobson, 2004), it has become an increasingly significant aspect of advertising claims and other promotional strategies. Children appear to have more influence over the purchase of food, holidays, hardware (such as electrical goods) and gifts for friends and family, although they are less influential in respect of larger investments such as cars and property. Girls have more influence in the purchasing of gifts, while boys play a more important role in choices of electrical goods, music and games (SIRC, 2009b). This influence can extend from initiating purchases to collecting information on alternatives, or suggesting retailers. Although it is extremely difficult to quantify, this 'influence market' is economically much more significant than the children's market per se (McNeal, 1999).

This growing significance of children as economic actors within the family reflects ideological changes as well as material ones. As we have seen (chapter 4), there has been a broader historical shift in beliefs about child rearing, towards a much more egalitarian approach. There has been a growing emphasis on the need for negotiation, openness and dialogue between parents and children, rather than the mere imposition of parental authority (Lee, 2001). What might be termed 'pedagogic' parenting has become the socially acceptable norm, although childcare advisers are often keen to distinguish this from the merely permissive variety (e.g. Brown, 2006).

This has in turn been manifested in changing approaches to family spending. Marketing researchers typically find that parents today are more likely to consult children about such matters than they were in earlier times. Indeed, according to the leading authority on children's marketing, James McNeal (1999), the contemporary family is now a 'filarchy', in which much of the decision-making power has been ceded to children. Definitive evidence for this would be difficult to establish, but it would seem likely for several reasons. With more mothers working, tasks such as shopping may be more likely to fall to children. Partly through their exposure to advertising and marketing, children could well be seen to possess greater knowledge about purchasing and consumption. Indeed, it may be that in many areas (such as technology), children possess greater expertise than their parents, and can introduce them to new trends or products, contribute relevant information, and help them to install or use new products. This can also relieve parents of complex and time-consuming decision-making. This 'consultancy' role appears to be particularly important among mid- to late-teenagers, who often play a key part in family purchasing decisions in particular areas. Teenagers can mobilize knowledge gained from personal and friends' experiences, and from the internet and other media sources, as a means of exercising influence, and this is generally perceived in a positive way by parents (Ekstrom, 2007). Even so, children may be less influential, particularly in the final stages of decision-making and in relation to 'big ticket' purchases, than they aspire to be. As we shall see in the following section, while some regard children's growing influence here as entirely legitimate, others perceive it as a source of conflict and unhappiness that urgently needs to be addressed.

Investigating 'pester power': effects research

The notion of 'pester power' (or what is occasionally termed 'the nag factor') is routinely acknowledged on both sides of this debate. While marketers are understandably wary of such terms, most are inclined to celebrate what they see as children's increasing autonomy and their greater say in family decision-making (e.g. Sutherland and Thompson, 2001). By contrast, for campaigners, 'pester power' represents a further instance of the unwarranted intrusion of commercial forces into intimate family relationships. In fact, both in the UK and across Europe, regulation prohibits marketers from overtly encouraging children to pester their parents for purchases: the famous 1950s advertising slogan 'don't forget the Fruit Gums, mum!' would be proscribed under current legislation.[2] However, the invocation of 'pester power' does not need to be as direct as this: children today are not assumed to need explicit tutoring in order to make their consumer desires known. Yet to what extent is 'pester power' an apt or useful means of characterizing the relationships between parents, children and commercial marketers? Are children's purchasing requests simply an unwelcome and irritating source of family conflict? Are parents bound automatically to resist them? And where, ultimately, does the power lie in this relationship?

Much of the research on this issue has been conducted within the paradigm of 'media effects' (see chapter 3). While most of this work dates back to the 1970s (see John, 1999, for a review), over the past decade the Dutch researcher Moniek Buijzen and her colleagues have conducted a series of studies looking at the consequences for family life of children's exposure to television advertising. Buijzen's work focuses on what she terms the 'unintended effects' of advertising: the intended effect of increasing children's purchasing requests is seen to result in a range of unintended consequences, including increased family conflict, materialistic values, 'life dissatisfaction' and feelings of unhappiness and disappointment (Buijzen and Valkenburg, 2003). These consequences appear to be more acute for younger children, whose lack of knowledge and experience is believed to render them more vulnerable to persuasion. As a result of their inability to delay gratification and their tendency to use less sophisticated techniques in seeking to persuade parents, this is seen to lead in turn to greater conflict within the family.

The evidence for these claims, however, is rather limited. In common with many media effects researchers, Buijzen persistently represents correlations or associations between variables as though they constituted proof of causal connections. For example, Buijzen and Valkenburg (2003: 498–9) claim that 'advertising enhances materialism', although in fact their research shows only that children who watch more television are more likely to profess materialistic attitudes. The same confusion is apparent in their misleading claims that 'advertising causes parent–child conflict' and that it 'leads to disappointment and life dissatisfaction'. Of course, it may be that watching television advertising prompts children to pester their parents to buy things; but it may equally be that children who are inclined to do so anyway are more likely to pay close attention to advertising. It may also be that children who are inclined to get into conflicts with their parents (about purchases, or in general) also tend to watch more television. Clearly, the causal relationships could go in either direction; and it is very likely that other factors might influence both phenomena.[3] Poverty, for example, might well play a crucial role here: children in poorer households tend to watch more television, not least because they have fewer alternatives, and their requests for purchases may be more likely to result in conflict if there is less money to go around.

In subsequent studies, Buijzen and her colleagues have explored the ways in which parents might 'mediate' the effects of advertising – although the term 'mediation' again implies that parents should act as a kind of barrier or filter in a process that is essentially one of cause-and-effect. The research here distinguishes between two forms of mediation: 'active' mediation entails talking to your children about what they watch, while 'restrictive' mediation involves attempting to reduce their exposure. These forms are related to broader patterns of family communication: 'concept-oriented' families are more inclined to discuss and negotiate, while in 'socio-oriented' families there is a greater emphasis on obedience and agreement (Buijzen and Valkenburg, 2005). In subsequent studies, comparisons are made between 'factual' mediation (for example, informing children about the persuasive intentions of advertising or about media techniques) and 'evaluative' mediation (for example, simply dismissing or rejecting advertising claims). These different forms of mediation are seen to create cognitive or attitudinal 'defences' against the influence of advertising (Buijzen, 2007, 2009; Buijzen and Mens, 2007).

Some of the latter research is experimental (e.g. Buijzen and Mens, 2007). For instance, children in a classroom are shown a three-minute tape of six commercials, followed by an experimenter making comments; and they are then subjected to a twenty-minute battery of test questions designed to assess the effectiveness of the different forms of commentary (for example, in terms of whether children say they are more or less likely to ask their parents for the products advertised). Such research is clearly unlikely to provide much insight into how parents and children behave in real life. The findings of this work are also contradictory. For instance, while one diary-based study finds that a socio-oriented approach is more effective (Buijzen, 2009), another suggests that a concept-oriented approach works best (Buijzen and Valkenburg, 2005). In some cases, younger children appear more likely to be influenced by factual mediation rather than evaluative, while the opposite seems to be the case with older children – an unexpected finding that points to the rather arbitrary distinction between factual and evaluative in the first place (Buijzen, 2007).

Criticisms might also be raised of some of the theoretical constructs that are employed in this kind of work, and how they are measured. 'Materialism', for example, is defined in the literature in a wide range of ways; various different scales are employed to measure it; and, as a result, the findings of such research are inconsistent and sometimes quite contradictory (see chapter 9). The distinction between 'socio-oriented' and 'concept-oriented' families is highly value-laden, and seems to consider 'communication style' as a fixed variable that can be considered in isolation from other social and material dimensions of family life.[4] Both these qualities are assessed by means of reports of attitudes or behaviour, which means they are very likely to be affected by 'social desirability' biases: people in certain social groups, or of particular ages, may be more or less likely to produce 'politically correct' responses. Meanwhile, children are understood here in terms of a deficit model, and defined as essentially incompetent: they are judged in terms of what they *cannot* do, rather than what they actually do – while adults or parents are assumed to be automatically capable of making rational judgements and decisions. The model of the family here is implicitly parent-centric: parents are positioned as moderators or controllers of their children's consumer desires, rather than in any sense participants in consumer culture themselves.

Above all, however, it is the fundamental notion of 'effects' that is most problematic here. Once again, it is assumed that people's relationships with consumer culture can be reduced to a series of cause-and-effect equations, and that these can be simply extracted out from other aspects of their social lives. Children's purchasing requests are implicitly seen to derive primarily from advertising, while parenting is reduced to a matter of more or less effective policing of consumption – as though parents were somehow external to the process, or merely a kind of variable in the equation. Mediation is seen to create psychological 'defences' that can apparently serve to insulate children from the effects of advertising – an approach that provides a highly simplistic way of understanding how people interpret and use marketing communications (see chapter 3).

'Pester power': alternative approaches

Catriona Nash (2009) provides an important critique of the notion of 'pester power', arguing that it offers a very narrow account of what she calls 'parent–child purchase relationships'. As she suggests, 'pester power' is itself a pejorative concept: it implies that children's purchasing requests are unwelcome, and that they necessarily involve persistent forms of whining and moaning that parents are bound to find exasperating. Yet children have limited disposable income, rare opportunities to shop independently, and may lack the ability to articulate their wants and needs in ways that adults find acceptable. As such, 'pestering' (or rather requesting parents to make purchases) is inevitable. Reviewing a wide range of previous research, Nash finds that children pragmatically adopt a range of strategies in requesting purchases, few of which entail anything that might be defined as 'pestering'. Likewise, parents' responses do not suggest that such requests frequently result in conflict, or that they are mostly annoying or exasperating, and few children seem disappointed by their parents' refusals. Significantly, a relatively small proportion of such requests appear to be caused or prompted by advertising, and advertising declines in significance as children get older.

Some recent empirical research provides support for this account. In Nash's own study, which uses qualitative interviews, her Irish respondents present this as a 'game' whose rules are well understood, and as a natural and expected part of family interaction. Parents and children aim to strike a balance here: parents sometimes accede to their children's requests, and sometimes avoid, distract or stall them, as well as refusing outright, while children make careful judgements about the types and the timing of their requests, and the strategies they use with different parents. Children, she argues, are generally accepting of their parents' authority, and understand their financial pressures. The overall picture that emerges here is not of families riven by conflict, unhappiness and materialistic attitudes (as in the media effects research discussed above), but rather of a knowing and playful approach on both sides. This is a game in which advertising is a relatively minor player: family and peers are much more significant influences.

Similar findings emerge from studies of shopping that use observational methods. For example, a couple of recent Danish studies have observed how children's influence 'plays out' in family supermarket shopping. Maria Norgaard and Karen Brunso (2010) find that a wide range of considerations and negotiations are involved in food purchasing, including the tastes and preferences of different family members; knowledge about nutrition and food preparation; judgements about quantity, quality and value for money; willingness to try new products; and estimates of family need. Likewise, Marlene Gram (2010) finds that decision-making involves a complex range of negotiating strategies: decisions are often made very quickly, and while they are sometimes democratically agreed, they are not always carefully considered or consistent. It is not always clear who influences whom in this process: children are not always on the side of emotion or desire, while parents are not always on the side of rationality.

In a different context, Christine Williams's (2006) ethnography of US toy stores makes similar observations about the negotiations between parents and children. In this case, parents may seek to teach their children the rules of thrifty shopping, or encourage them to choose products that carry greater cultural capital, although they also seek to gratify the child's desires. Perhaps a little facetiously, Williams suggests that there is an element of 'sado-masochism' in this process. Parents typically buy toys for their children as special treats or rewards for good behaviour, but bringing them into a toy store conveys a mixed message: controlling your desires, being 'good', will eventually enable you to 'splurge' and give in to temptation. Children may develop fears that they are not loved if they do not receive gifts, while parents may worry that children are only well behaved because they want more toys. As this implies, the emotional dimensions of shopping can prove highly ambivalent, on the part of parents as well as children.

Meanwhile, a couple of recent UK studies have explored the range of criteria that are at play in how parents respond to children's purchasing requests. Julie Evans and Joan Chandler (2006) find that parents take account of value for money, educational qualities and the longer-term potential for enjoyment and use of particular products, as well as the persistence with which children make requests; while Sharon Boden (2006a) finds that in the case of children's clothing, parents consider factors such as quality, value for money and age-appropriateness as well as branding. A range of other issues is raised in these studies that begin to point to some of the complexities at stake. For example, Evans and Chandler find that parents are especially sensitive to their children's desire to 'fit in' with their peers (an issue that will be considered in the next chapter), and that they will look back to their own childhoods in attempting to make sense of their children's consumer desires. Meanwhile, Boden finds that children can influence their parents' tastes in clothing, helping to 'modernize' their personal style – a form of 'reverse socialization' that also applies in areas such as technology and media consumption (see chapter 3). Like Williams (2006), Evans and Chandler make the crucial point that buying can also entail and express complex feelings of love, intimacy and guilt.

All these studies focus primarily on the negotiations that surround the actual purchasing of goods. Yet, as I have argued, 'consumption' is also about the use and circulation of products beyond this point. In this respect, the negotiations between parents and children considered in chapters 6 and 7 – about what to eat and what to wear – are also relevant here, as are the broader anthropological studies of consumption discussed in chapter 2. These studies, along with some to be considered in the next section of this chapter, provide an alternative to the rather bleak image of family conflict that is offered by the media effects research. They also suggest that advertising – or marketing more broadly – is a relatively insignificant influence in this respect. Furthermore, they show that parents' roles in relation to children's consumption are much more complex than a simple matter of 'mediation'. On the contrary, parents may accede to their children's requests not because of some perceived inability to resist the 'power' of advertising, but rather because of their own emotional investments in consumption.

As this implies, parents are often complicit in children's consumption, rather than being merely external regulators. Parents buy things for their children as an expression of love and care, and of wanting to please and delight – and this is another facet of parents' emotional life to which marketers have consistently sought to appeal (Cross, 2004). Yet these emotions may also be quite ambivalent, and even contradictory. They are often tied up with parents' feelings of guilt and anxiety, with fantasies and projections about childhood, and with concerns about their own and their children's social status.

Thus, as we have seen, contemporary parents are experiencing a growing sense of 'time pressure': spending less time with their children than they believe they should, they invest more heavily in it, both emotionally and financially. Consulting with children about purchasing, and being more inclined to accede to their demands, can thus be seen to provide a form of compensation for parental guilt or anxiety. At the same time, 'indulging' one's children can also represent an attempt to come to terms with the loss of one's own childhood; and there may be a tension between parents' desire to shelter and nurture their children and their wish to allow children a space for self-expression, in which they can enjoy the freedom they themselves have lost (Cross, 2010). Social mobility may also play a role here: upwardly mobile parents may seek to provide children with goods that they were 'denied' in their own childhood; yet they may also feel uneasy about the contrast between their own childhood experiences (often idealistically recalled as consumption-free) and those of their own children. In this way, the past may become implicated with the present and with the future, as parents also look to their children to realize their own unfulfilled aspirations.

Meanwhile, children can also serve as vehicles for parental consumption, and particularly for the conspicuous display of high-status goods, well before they are able to articulate their own wants or needs. Research in more wealthy societies such as Norway has pointed to the phenomenon of 'trophy children', and the considerable amounts of money spent on items such as high-tech buggies (strollers), designer baby clothes and play equipment by affluent parents, and indeed grandparents (Brusdal, 2008). Similar tendencies are apparent in the rise of the designer childrenswear market, to be discussed in the following chapter (Crewe and Collins, 2006). Meanwhile, as we shall see in chapter 11, marketers also target parents through appealing to beliefs about good parenting, not least in selling educational goods and services. In this sense, children's consumption can serve as a proxy or vehicle for parents' displays of material and cultural capital – or alternatively as evidence of the lack of it (cf. Bourdieu, 1979).

Inequality and the contradictions of care

These latter points are explored in considerable detail in Allison Pugh's remarkable ethnographic study of US families, *Longing and Belonging* (2009). Pugh's central concern is with the ways in which commercial forces connect with the social meanings surrounding parental care. As she suggests, this plays out in very different ways across social classes. For the most part, the affluent parents in her study are highly ambivalent about their children's involvement in consumer culture. They struggle to restrain their children's consumer desires, for example by means of rules and allowances; they eschew conspicuous consumption in favour of 'symbolic deprivation'; and in some instances express considerable disdain for children's tastes and for commercial values more broadly.[5] Yet many of these parents are themselves upwardly mobile, and experienced feelings of deprivation in their own childhood, and, as a result, they seek to give their children 'the things they never had', sponsoring their consumption even as they attempt to restrict it. By contrast, the low-income parents are less ambivalent. They are highly sensitive to their children's feelings of exclusion from the peer group, and seek to protect them from the stigma of poverty by providing them with high-status clothing and branded goods. They regard buying things for their children as an unequivocal sign of 'good parenting', and do not express moral qualms about the quantity of possessions their children have. However, due to the cyclical and insecure nature of low-wage employment, their ability to provide for their children is more intermittent: periods of constraint alternate with periods of 'symbolic indulgence' or 'windfall child rearing', and such parents often go without in order to buy things for their children.

Pugh's study moves beyond the easy polarization that we have seen in previous chapters, between the view of children as dupes of marketers and the celebration of creative consumption. However, she is highly critical of what she regards as the 'commodification of difference, care and belonging'. As she argues, children's consumer desires stem less from vulnerability to commercial persuasion than from the emotional values that are associated with consumer goods (which do not derive simply from advertising). Albeit in different ways, the parents in her study also appear to be highly susceptible to the idea that the nature and extent of their 'provisioning' – what they buy (or do not buy) for their children – is a significant indicator of their love and care. Yet, to some extent, parents are also merely bystanders in their children's attempts to find belonging and inclusion within the peer group. They are highly sensitive to what Pugh calls the 'economy of dignity' within the peer group – the sense that status is dependent upon the display of consumer goods and consumer knowledge. (This latter aspect will be considered more fully in the following chapter.) Both for parents and children, she argues, care and belonging have come to be mediated – and to some extent defined – through market relations, and this is a phenomenon that ultimately reinforces social inequality.

As Pugh also suggests, consumption is not simply a matter of the acquisition of goods, but also of experiences – not least 'educational' experiences. Middle-class parents are in a better position to purchase the social contexts in which children's childhoods take place – neighbourhoods, schools and other forms of childcare, as well as holidays and out-of-school activities – and may well prioritize this over the accumulation of 'stuff'. The different 'pathways' parents are able to buy for their children thereby further reinforce segregation and inequality.

Pugh's findings here are informed and confirmed by a previous ethnographic study, Annette Lareau's *Unequal Childhoods* (2003). Although Lareau is not directly concerned with the role of consumption, she does consider the economic dimensions of parenting across different social classes. Lareau identifies a form of middle-class parenting that she calls 'concerted cultivation' – a hectic and expensive schedule of piano and ballet lessons, private tutoring, organized sports and other 'improving' experiences that Valerie Walkerdine (1999) has elsewhere described as the 'full diary syndrome'. As Lareau (2003) suggests, this purposeful attempt to develop their talents and aspirations breeds 'a robust sense of entitlement' among middle-class children, which may also result in escalating demands on their exhausted parents. By contrast, she finds that working-class children are more likely to be left alone to manage their own time, along with peers – an approach she terms 'the accomplishment of natural growth'. However, the less structured and parentally supervised leisure experiences of working-class children may render them less amenable to the discipline of school and other institutionalized settings, and hence less likely to achieve. As Lareau makes clear, these different approaches to child rearing depend very much on the economic resources available: the expenditure involved, for instance in attending organized sports activities, was often considered negligible by more affluent parents but was a formidable constraint for poor families. Yet this is not simply a matter of different opportunities for spending time: what wealthy parents are uniquely positioned to do here is (in Bourdieu's terms) to convert economic capital into cultural capital, and to develop a set of dispositions that are likely to ensure future success. Children, in this sense, are very much seen as investments for the future.

There is also some striking evidence on these class differences from research in the UK. Carol Vincent and Stephen Ball (2007) provide an analysis of what they call the 'making up' of the middle-class child that has much in common with Lareau's account of 'concerted cultivation'. They describe the extensive range of commercially provided 'enrichment' activities (such as sports, arts and foreign language classes) that affluent middle-class parents are increasingly purchasing for their pre-school-aged children. Such provision is supported by the proliferating amount of advice literature (for example in the form of glossy parenting magazines), which stresses the need for parents to secure 'learning readiness' and to provide a 'creative environment' for their children. As Vincent and Ball suggest, 'the child here is understood as a project – soft, malleable and able to be developed and improved' (p. 1065). Also following Bourdieu (1979), they argue that these activities serve to develop particular tastes and dispositions that are seen as markers of social status; and, as such, they can be seen as a strategy designed to reproduce existing patterns of social inequality. In some instances, the parents in their study appeared to be using such activities as a means of starting to build their child's CV (or résumé) in preparation for competitive entry to selective schools at the age of 11. Here again, parents appear to feel an urgent sense of obligation to provide the maximum opportunities for their child's capacities to develop to the full; and, as Vincent and Ball suggest, this may be intensifying as a result of social changes, in which the future success of middle-class children can no longer be so easily secured (a phenomenon also identified in the US context by Ehrenreich, 1990).

By contrast, Tess Ridge (2002) has studied the negotiations around money and expenditure that occur in 'socially excluded' or poor families. Among her sample, only a minority of children were regularly receiving pocket money; and, of those who were, some were using it as means to pay for necessities such as clothing and transport to school. Although some were able to supplement their income through working, their lack of resources generated considerable difficulties in terms of their status and sense of inclusion within the peer group (an issue to be considered in the following chapter). They were often unable to participate in commercially provided leisure activities, and few families could afford holidays. However, these children showed a complex understanding of their parents' financial constraints. When they needed their parents to buy something for them, they would adjust their expectations, or simply not ask, in light of economic circumstances. There is evidence here of poor parents attempting to protect their children from the stigma of poverty, for example by going without purchases themselves in order to provide their children with high-status items of clothing (see also Gordon et al., 2006; Middleton et al., 1998). However, there are also instances of children (especially girls) attempting to protect their parents, moderating their demands in order to avoid causing additional stress (cf. Chin, 2001). Yet when asked what they would change about their lives, these children did not express a wish for more expensive possessions, but rather for more opportunities to socialize with friends, or for some relief from their everyday personal struggles.

There is undoubtedly a danger in some of these studies of unduly polarizing 'middle-class' and 'working-class' experiences, and of ignoring the more mundane phenomena – including commercial phenomena – that constitute the 'common culture' of childhood. Family life entails a whole range of everyday experiences, rituals and routines that are common to all. Despite some parents' attempts to micro-manage their children's time, and some children's exclusion from participation, most children have access to aspects of commercial media and marketing that are shared across all social classes. Furthermore, it could be argued that for all parents, the fundamental experience here is one of ambivalence. Even wealthy parents, who may be able to buy their children everything they want and need (and more), appear to regard consumer culture with a degree of guilt, regret and uncertainty; and while such parents may spend a great deal of time and money on 'cultivating' their children, they are generally aware of the risks of 'hot-housing' them, and of their need to relax and have fun outside of adult supervision. Nevertheless, there remain striking inequalities in children's experiences of family life, and in their engagements with consumer culture, and this issue will therefore be pursued further in the following chapters.

Conclusion

Before concluding this chapter, it should be acknowledged that my account here has been largely gender-blind. Yet much of the debate about parents' role in children's consumption is implicitly about *mothers*. Most of the research I have considered notes the fact that it is mothers rather than fathers who are typically seen to be responsible for managing or overseeing children's consumption: it is mothers who seem to be best placed to know what children want, and who do most of the actual buying (see, among others, Evans and Chandler, 2006; Nash, 2009; Pugh, 2009; Vincent and Ball, 2007). Equally, within the popular debate, it is typically mothers who are accused of being 'bad consumers' and of failing to regulate their children's desires: as in so many areas, it is predominantly mothers who are blamed for problems with children's development or socialization. Yet the gendering of this relationship is rarely addressed in any explicit way, and it remains an issue that urgently needs to be taken up in future research.

In this chapter, I have attempted to illustrate the value of a 'relational' approach to children's consumption, which locates it in a wider network of social relationships. As I have argued, parents are implicated in a whole variety of ways here. Yet, while they continue to play a crucial role, peers become increasingly important as children grow older – and, as many of the studies I have discussed clearly show, parents often perceive their own power to be highly contingent upon what they sometimes describe as 'peer pressure' (e.g. Pugh, 2009; Ridge, 2002). It is accordingly to this issue that I turn in the following chapter.

9

Beyond 'peer pressure'

Consumption and identity in the peer group

Parents and marketers are, of course, not the only significant players in children's consumption. From the moment they begin to interact with each other, children express and display their own consumer preferences. Their first tentative engagements with other children in the playground or the nursery often focus on the manipulation of toys or tools that are, for the most part, commercial products. Finding and maintaining the common ground that is necessary for play depends upon the agreement of shared meanings that are at least partly drawn from consumer culture. As children get older, what they wear, what they eat, what they play with – or refuse to wear or eat or play with – is increasingly subject to negotiation with their peers. By the time they come to spend their own disposable income, children's primary point of reference is much more likely to be the desires and preferences of other children than those of their parents.

As we have seen, many parents are highly attuned to their children's need to find acceptance within the peer group. 'Peer pressure' is frequently perceived as a key influence on children's requests for purchases, and is often seen to possess an irresistible force. Evans and Chandler (2006), for example, describe parents feeling they have to surrender to peer pressure, not least in order to avoid their children being teased or bullied. The youngest children in their study (aged 7) were very aware of the need to 'fit in' with friends and the possibility of being marginalized if they wore the 'wrong' clothes or failed to buy in to the latest consumer 'fads'. Peer group norms – in terms of dress and appearance, but also media, toys and other consumer goods – are often seen to override the wishes and values of parents; and of course for many parents this is an exasperating reminder of the limitations of their own power and authority.

Allison Pugh's (2009) research, discussed in chapter 8, particularly focuses on what she calls the 'economy of dignity' that operates among peers. For example, she explores how children (as young as first grade) engage in forms of 'facework' or impression management in order to achieve belonging within the peer group. Access to consumer culture – owning or merely knowing about key aspects of media, toys, and other merchandise – provides a key means of establishing status and acceptance. This is to some extent taken as evidence of parental 'provisioning': children's efforts to show that they are sufficiently cared-for result in constant competition over the amount and value of their possessions. Yet it is also to some extent independent of, and even resistant towards, the values of parents: for example, demonstrating insider knowledge of 'adult' television programmes – or disavowing interest in ones that are deemed to be 'childish' – can be a powerful means of establishing one's status as 'cool' and hence as 'popular'. Yet this process is subject to continual negotiation – claiming and counter-claiming, concealing and disavowing, patrolling and disciplining: in the cut-and-thrust of children's interactions, inclusion within a given friendship group is always insecure and provisional.

Social inequalities are certainly apparent in Pugh's research. The more affluent children were inclined to boast of different things – such as foreign holidays or pricier venues for family outings or birthday parties – while the poorer children were more subject to the vicissitudes of 'windfall child rearing'. Different 'tokens of dignity' also carried different amounts of value in different social and institutional settings, not least as schools attempted to prevent children from bringing in particular types of products. Nevertheless, commercial goods served as a shared form of symbolic language for children from all backgrounds here. Ultimately, Pugh argues that – like relationships of care between parents and children – children's peer group relationships have been permeated by market culture: consumption has become central to social inclusion, and money has effectively been equated with belonging (2009: 51).

Yet to what extent is this rather baleful conclusion corroborated by other research? Does 'who you are' now depend simply on 'what you can buy'? Do commercial influences in some way intensify the competitive pressure of children's peer groups, or would such pressure exist in any case? Are children and parents merely victims of 'peer pressure' – and, indeed, is 'peer pressure' a useful means of conceptualizing the role of consumption in children's social relationships? This chapter begins by looking at the question of social identity and its relationship to children's consumption. It then moves on to look at the area of media consumption; and, in more detail, at clothing and fashion. Finally, it returns more directly to the broader question of 'materialism', and the recurring claim that possessions have now become more important to us than people.

Consumption, social identity and childhood

Various theories have been used to explain the role of social identity in children's consumption. Psychologists argue that the influence of parents diminishes as children become increasingly involved in the wider social world, and particularly in the peer group. They typically see this as a necessary developmental stage in the emergence of a well-adjusted adult identity (e.g. Erikson, 1968; Howe, 2010). Likewise, in 'consumer socialization' research, children are seen to move towards a final, 'reflective' stage in which the social meanings of consumption come to the fore (John, 1999). Thus, in the early teenage years, children increasingly make judgements about people on the basis of their consumer preferences, and use products to communicate their own personal style and identity. This is seen to be a function of their cognitive development – their growing ability to engage in 'perspective taking' (seeing the world from others' point of view) and 'social comparison'. It also relates to their social development, and the learning of skills such as personal interaction, collaboration, and dealing with conflict. However, as we have seen (chapter 3), there are some significant problems with these kinds of developmental models – not least, in this case, the fact that such complex negotiations with peers are apparent among much younger children (cf. Corsaro, 1997).

More sociological theories of identity have addressed these issues in different ways. Broadly speaking, the emphasis here is on the social processes whereby individuals seek to define themselves as members of groups. 'Social identity theory', for example, is concerned with the ways in which people construct 'in group' and 'out group' relationships: it explores processes such as social comparison, inclusion and exclusion, categorization and stereotyping (R. Jenkins, 2004). Poststructuralist approaches explore similar issues in terms of how individuals 'position' themselves and others, or how social identities are 'performed' in particular settings or relationships (Hall, 1992). What these theories have in common is a sense of the construction of identity, not as a singular achievement (that might be attained on reaching adulthood, for example), but rather as a process of ongoing work. Identity is not singular or given, but rather multiple, shifting and always incomplete; and it is not an internal possession, but rather something that is socially negotiated and achieved in specific settings. In a sense, the process might more appropriately be seen not in terms of 'identity' (a fixed object) but rather in terms of 'identification' (a process): identity here is something you *do* rather than something you *are*.

(Overviews of these theories, albeit more in relation to youth than to children, may be found in Buckingham, 2008b, and Phoenix, 2009.)

From this perspective, consumer culture is seen to provide symbolic resources that people use to communicate and make meaning, and thereby to signify or make claims about their identity. For Anthony Giddens (1991), for example, consumer culture provides at least part of the means by which people reflexively construct identity: it is a key dimension of what he calls 'the project of the self'. As we have seen (chapter 2), 'postmodernist' theories make much of the ways in which consumers actively create and express individual identity through their consumer choices and practices. Clothing, for example, has been seen to provide a system of social meanings that consumers may use to define aspects of their social identity, and to engage in a (sometimes playful) performance of the self (see Craik, 2009). However, such theories tend to be highly individualistic: they are frequently criticized for failing to address the structuring influences of the market, and for presenting consumers as wholly autonomous. Here again, what seems to be needed is an approach that takes account of the fundamentally *relational* nature of consumption, and of children's consumption in particular.

Even so, these kinds of arguments do provide us with some useful ways of understanding the role of consumption in children's social relationships. They focus attention on how children seek to establish social status, how they present themselves and make judgements about other people, how they align themselves with others or seek to distance themselves from them, and how they seek to establish their own independence. They also alert us to what is a fundamental tension underlying many young people's accounts of identity, between the desire to affiliate and belong to the group and the desire to assert individual autonomy – or, in everyday terms, between 'fitting in' and 'standing out' (see, for example, Miles et al., 1998; Milner, 2004).

Why does consumer culture appear to occupy such a central role in this process? Murray Milner (2004) provides an interesting suggestion here, in the context of a detailed ethnographic study of the operation of peer groups in US high schools – a world of exclusive and competitive cliques made familiar around the world, but also sharply satirized, by movies such as *Mean Girls* (dir. Mark Waters, 2004). Milner argues that in contemporary US society, adolescents have considerable autonomy but little real economic or political power. They are segregated in institutions like schools, over which they have little control; and in many other areas of their lives, they are routinely humiliated and treated as inferior. The only real power they do have, he suggests, is in their evaluations of each other: they have 'the power to create status systems based on their own criteria' (p. 25) – and when 'left to their own devices' they are bound to turn to consumer culture for the resources with which to do so. Milner's research therefore traces how these high school students use the symbols, logos and products of the commercial market as means of claiming and marking out status hierarchies: the possession and display of goods (from clothing to music to mobile phones) serves to define social power and solidarity, to impose conformity to the norms of the group, and to express resistance to adult authority.

Milner's account is based on a relatively unfashionable theoretical source, Max Weber's theory of status groups, although (at least in respect of consumption) it has much in common with the work of Bourdieu, discussed in chapter 2. His account of status hierarchies could be accused of being unduly deterministic: most young people are not members of the narrowly defined cliques he identifies, even if they may be influenced by them; and other research suggests that, at least in more socially diverse, multicultural settings, there may be multiple hierarchies and competing standards of value in operation (Pomerantz, 2008). Milner's proposals that schools should employ various means of excluding consumer culture and thereby preventing social competition (such as uniforms, or the random assignment of students to classes) seem to require schools to operate as 'total institutions' with absolute control over their inmates. Yet, despite these criticisms, he does provide an explanation of the role of consumer culture that moves beyond a view of young people as merely victims of manipulative marketing, or indeed as products of poor parenting. Rather, according to Milner, it is the structure of the education system which keeps young people confined to the peer group, and results in their preoccupation with status; and it is this in turn that contributes to their preoccupation with consumer culture, and hence to the creation and maintenance of consumer capitalism.[1]

Media talk and the negotiation of identity

Research on children's consumption of media provides some significant support for this approach. In my own work, I have looked in considerable detail at the shifting social dynamics that are at play in children's talk about television and other media (e.g. Buckingham, 1993a, c, 1996, 2000b; Buckingham and Bragg, 2004). The focus here has been on how children's talk about media functions as a form of 'identity work'. In staking out their tastes and preferences, and proclaiming and debating their judgements about media, children are simultaneously making claims about their own identities. From this perspective, talk comes to be seen not as some kind of self-evident reflection of what children 'really' think or believe, but rather as a form of social action or performance (cf. Potter and Wetherell, 1987). Children's judgements about genre and representation, or their retellings of film or television narratives, are analysed here not as cognitive processes but as inherently social actions; and the development of knowledge about media ('media literacy') is seen in terms of their social motivations and purposes.

For example, I have focused in several studies on children's use of 'critical' discourses about television, and their functions in terms of social identity (Buckingham, 1993a, c). Thus, boys' talk about soap operas – and their judgements about what is or is not realistic or plausible – is inextricably related to their ongoing construction of their own masculinity, while girls' frequent complaints about the 'unrealistic' storylines or events in action-adventure cartoons often reflect a desire to distance themselves from what are seen as boys' 'childish' tastes, and thereby to proclaim their own (gendered) maturity. Boys' rejection of melodrama or girls' rejection of violent action movies can thus be seen as rather more than the mechanical application of fixed judgements of taste: on the contrary, they represent an active *claim* to a particular social position – a claim which is sometimes tentative and uncertain, and in many cases open to challenge.

Furthermore, such judgements may also play a role in enabling viewers retrospectively to regulate or indeed disclaim their own *affective* responses – for example, of fear or sorrow. Speculating about the special effects in horror films, or condemning them as 'unrealistic', for instance, may serve to preclude the accusation that one might be 'soft' enough to find them frightening, and appears to be a particular preoccupation for some boys. While the pleasure of such films clearly must depend to some extent upon the willing 'suspension of disbelief' – in effect, on consenting to let yourself be frightened – this kind of subsequent discussion can serve as a means of learning how to 'handle' potentially unwelcome emotional reactions, and of projecting a more 'adult' identity (Buckingham, 1996).

This approach moves beyond a view of meaning-making as merely a psychological phenomenon, which happens 'inside children's heads'. On the contrary, this kind of critical talk is seen to serve particular social or interpersonal functions in the context of dialogue with others. The context of the research itself is clearly crucial here. Any adult asking children questions about television – particularly in a school context, as has generally been the case in my research – is likely to invite these critical discourses. Most children know that many adults disapprove of them watching 'too much' television, and they are familiar with at least some of the arguments about its negative effects upon them. In some instances, these arguments are addressed directly, although children are generally keen to exempt themselves from such charges: while their younger siblings might copy what they watch, such accusations certainly do not apply to *them*. Just as adults appear to displace the 'effects' of television onto children – thereby implying that they themselves are not at risk – so children tend to suggest that these arguments only apply to those much younger than themselves.

In a sense, judgements about the 'unreality' of television could be seen to serve a similar function, albeit in a more indirect way. They enable the speaker to present him- or herself as a sophisticated viewer, who is able to 'see through' the illusions television provides. In effect, they represent a claim for social status – and, particularly in this context, a claim to be 'adult'. While these claims may be at least partly directed towards the interviewer and towards other children in the group, they often seem to rely on distinguishing the speaker from an invisible 'other' – from those viewers who are immature or stupid enough to believe that what they watch is real. In this respect, talk about television can also function as a means of performing or making claims about age identities, or of 'generationing' (see chapter 3).

This research has largely been conducted in the context of focus groups; yet, in many respects, it would seem to reflect at least some of what occurs in more naturalistic settings. Recent research in schools using 'eavesdropping' techniques (including radio microphones) has reported numerous instances of children incorporating media references in their everyday interactions in the playground or on the margins of classroom activities (Dover, 2007; Rampton et al., 2002). Here again, the display of 'expert' knowledge, tastes and enthusiasms in everyday chat can serve as a means of defining one's identity and position within the peer group, and in relation to the 'official' culture of the school.

Participatory media and branded identities

This social construction of identity is equally apparent in young people's engagements with new digital media. As I have noted (chapter 5), companies are increasingly looking to more participatory 'Web 2.0' services such as social networking sites as vehicles for marketing – even if the commercial dimensions of these media are not always apparent to their users. Facilities such as Facebook are highly commercial spaces, both in the sense that they are commercially owned and operated, and in that they frequently serve as vehicles for marketing or for gathering information about consumers' habits and preferences. Such services make money partly by inserting commercial messages in the context of children's peer-group interactions – for example through competitions and quizzes using branded content. In the process, users also become targets for forms of embedded marketing, including viral and peer-to-peer marketing that appears to originate from individuals rather than from companies; the content they generate is often owned by the service provider; and their personal data can be harvested by marketers through online questionnaires and 'cookies' (Montgomery, 2007). More broadly, such services could be seen to encourage commercially defined constructions of identity: users are required to define themselves through their consumer preferences, and through specific acts of consumption; they are encouraged to use branded resources to design their personal profile pages, and to engage in communication with others; and they are effectively forced to 'advertise' and 'promote' themselves, or rather particular versions of themselves (Skaar, 2010).

Marketers and enthusiasts typically justify such activities on the grounds that they encourage 'participation', 'creativity' and 'self-expression'. Children here are no longer mere 'consumers': on the contrary, they effectively serve as the distributors or creators of commercial messages. This approach has a particularly compelling appeal for young people at an age where questions about personal identity formation and peer-group interaction represent a very prominent focus of concern. In these media, marketing is thus inextricably woven into children's social lives, and into their sense of themselves as autonomous social actors, to the point where it is hard to see how adults (parents or teachers) might intervene (Skaar et al., 2010).

To date, much of the debate in this area has focused only on more spectacular forms of 'cyber-bullying' (Brandtzaeg, 2009; Slonje and Smith, 2007) – although it can be hard to define what counts as 'bullying' in this context, or to identify how the particular characteristics of online media may exacerbate it. Yet there may be more significant and pervasive consequences of the use of online media in terms of how identities and relationships are coming to be defined and lived out (Ito et al., 2010). These media implicitly favour certain forms of self-representation and communication, and marginalize or exclude others; and these in turn may implicitly define what it means to be an individual, a person of a certain age or gender or social group, or indeed a 'friend'. Meanwhile, young people are also actively constructing their own social norms, conventions and forms of 'etiquette' in online spaces, which serve to sustain or erase boundaries, to regulate behaviour and to promote particular forms of identification. In the process, the meanings of individuality, identity and intimacy may change – and the risks of failure may be amplified or intensified.

These new media offer many new possibilities for the construction of identity, although they also pose new constraints and make possible new forms of regulation and surveillance. They provide new forms of play and sociability, but they do so in ways that are far from being as free or open – or indeed as liberating – as they may seem. Both online and offline, issues of inclusion and exclusion, and the establishment and negotiation of status hierarchies, are central preoccupations for young people. Online media may intensify or dramatize these processes, but the more spectacular risks need to be understood in the context of more mundane online behaviour.

Clothing: brands and markets

The role of consumption in the construction of children's social identity is even more apparent in the field of clothing. As I have noted, dress has been often seen to function as a kind of language through which we signify our individuality – and particularly our sense of belonging, ambivalence or resistance towards particular social groups or categories (Barthes, 1990; Lurie, 1983). Of course, this is partly driven by market forces – although it is by no means a recent development. In the case of children, Clare Rose (2010) has shown how rapid innovations in design – more in boys' clothing than in girls' – in the late nineteenth century were used to drive consumer demand, and she recounts incidents of how this in turn became a focus of competitiveness and bullying in the playground. In recent years, however, the emphasis appears to have shifted from clothing in general to brands more specifically: as brand names and logos have increasingly been on display on the clothing itself, brands themselves have come to be used as key signifiers – as means of making claims about one's own identity, and of judging others (Phoenix, 2009). Even so, the social meanings of brands are far from fixed; and there have been notable instances of clothing companies struggling to contain and prevent the circulation of 'unofficial' meanings surrounding certain brands – for example, when they become the focus of political campaigns (as in the case of Nike), or when the products are taken up by groups of consumers whom the manufacturers regard as socially undesirable (as in the case of Tommy Hilfiger or Burberry).

The children's clothing industry in the UK appears to have expanded fairly significantly in the 1990s, peaking at around £6 billion per year, although it has since declined somewhat.[2] Nevertheless, according to Crewe and Collins (2006), this sector has been largely transformed through a new focus on design, quality and style: childrenswear has increasingly become subject to the imperatives of fashion. As Boden (2006b) suggests, pop and sports celebrities have also come to play a vital role in defining the social meanings of particular clothing styles in the children's and youth market – not least by officially endorsing them, or in some cases actually 'designing' them. Here again, media – especially popular music and teen magazines – act as significant intermediaries in children's consumption.

However, this market also appears to have undergone a degree of polarization. On the one hand, we have seen the expansion of the market for 'designer' childrenswear: upmarket global brands such as Armani, Versace, DKNY and Prada have all created children's ranges, specialist magazines like *Vogue Bambini* have launched, while less populist 'niche' designers such as Paul Smith and Katherine Hamnett in the UK have sought to appeal to fashion-conscious upper-middle-class parents (Crewe and Collins, 2006). On the other hand, supermarkets are taking a growing proportion of children's market share, having doubled to almost 30 per cent of the market in the past five years.[3] According to de Kervenoael et al. (2008), this is partly about ease of access for shoppers (through linked grocery purchasing), as well as factors such as price, quality and value for money – although it is also a result of leading supermarkets seeking to establish their brands within this market, along with subsidiary ranges, celebrity endorsements and the growing use of online marketing. This has led to a situation in which supermarket clothing is no longer seen as 'throwaway' or taboo in fashion terms. As Pole et al. (2005) suggest, there has been a polarization here between 'generic' branding in supermarkets and high street chains, and 'independent' brands that are sold in a variety of outlets; and between 'top end' products and the 'value end' that is used for routine purchases. According to these authors, market research suggests that customers tend to use both types of products, depending upon the context. This would suggest that reports of the absolute victory of expensive 'designer' brands are far from true – and equally that parents and children are by no means as enslaved to such brands as they are sometimes accused of being.

Clothing, identity and inequality

Furthermore, this is not to imply that brands are equally important for all young people, or always in the same ways. While some studies report that girls are more 'fashion-conscious' than boys (Pole et al., 2005), others suggest that boys are more inclined to show an interest in brands per se (especially in relation to sportswear) than girls (Phoenix, 2009). While younger teenagers may have less disposable income, some research suggests that they are more interested in brands than older ones (Croghan et al., 2006). It should also be noted that there is resistance among some older young people to the prominence of brands, although of course this resistance might itself be seen as a form of statement about identity. More generally, most young people are keen to claim that they are by no means 'fashion victims' or 'followers of the crowd' (Phoenix, 2009): one of the most stigmatized identities among youth is the figure of the 'wannabee', the social outcast who tries too hard to gain entry to the group through the overt display of branded clothing.

Even so, there is ample evidence from research of the ways in which children use brands to mark out particular social identities, to define group norms, and to establish hierarchies of status. Gender is one key dimension here. For example, Jon Swain's (2002) ethnographic study describes how children in one working-class London primary school used clothing and footwear brands to seek recognition from peers, to generate common bonds, and to share intimacy. While groupings were flexible, inclusion in the dominant male groups depended very heavily on participation in sports, particular forms of speech and body language, and on the display of specific brands of sportswear – all of which contributed to the ongoing performance of 'cool'. The high-status boys in particular operated a hierarchy of brands, in which particular sports shoes had the greatest currency: Nike, above all, was taken to signify 'wealth, choice, freedom, equality, sportiness, casualness, anti-school, and ... collective belonging' (p. 61) – qualities that are of course directly promoted by Nike's own marketing. The price paid for such goods was crucial: it was important to make known that one had bought the shoes at full price in a 'real' shop rather than at a discount outlet. Those who conformed too closely to the school's (relatively flexible) uniform policy were often stigmatized and ridiculed as 'boffs' (that is, as too academic) or as 'gay' (a negative term, albeit one that did not necessarily imply any judgement about the wearer's sexuality). Wearing 'the right stuff' was a kind of cultural imperative, a proof of masculine competence – although not all the boys engaged in this struggle with equal commitment. Like Milner (2004), Swain suggests that these less affluent children had very few other means of claiming status available to them.

Swain's findings here are supported by a larger-scale UK study by Frosh et al. (2002), which notes the role of brands in defining and sustaining 'hegemonic masculinity' among older boys. Here again, boys could be ostracized for failing to wear the correct designer brands, and clothing was the focus for ongoing banter and 'jockeying for position' that is seen as characteristically male (cf. Buckingham, 1993c). However, Frosh et al. also find that this process is more prevalent among working-class boys: some of the upper-middle-class boys in their sample were disdainful of this focus on brands and designers (similar findings are reported in Bucholtz, 2007).

Shauna Pomerantz (2008) focuses on teenage girls, in a detailed ethnographic study set in a very diverse Vancouver high school – a study that (despite its different theoretical approach) has much in common with Milner's (2004) work on US high school cliques, discussed above. Here again, 'style' – in the form of clothing, but also hairstyles, bodily adornments and accessories – is seen to function as a kind of 'social skin', a means of communicating identity in social settings. Pomerantz traces how girls carefully select, customize and combine such elements in their efforts to position themselves in relation to intersecting categories of social identity (relating not only to gender, but also to age, social class and ethnicity). Here again, identity is only ever provisionally achieved: the girls have to work hard to attain legitimacy and authenticity, and, in particular, to avoid the stigmatized position of the overtly sexual 'skank'. Girls, she argues, adopt particular styles in attempting to be recognized as particular *kinds* of girls; but there is always a risk that they may be *mis*recognized, or positioned by others in ways that they do not wish. Pomerantz directly confronts popular claims about the 'sexualized' style of much contemporary girls' fashion (as discussed in relation to 'tweens' in chapter 7). While acknowledging that girls' identities are partly shaped by consumer culture, she challenges those who pathologize girls as dupes of marketing – whether in the form of ideas about 'false consciousness', or in more psychological claims that girls' attachment to brands is merely a symptom of their chronic lack of self-esteem, their conformism or their need for attention.

Richard Elliott and Clare Leonard (2004) draw out the social class dynamics here in a study of the consumption of sports shoes ('trainers') by less affluent children in the UK. Presented with a series of images of branded and non-branded shoes, the 8- to 12-year-olds in this study revealed a series of assumptions about their likely owners: those who wore expensive branded shoes were assumed to be wealthy and young, while those who wore inexpensive unbranded shoes would be poor and old. Children said they themselves were more likely to talk to people wearing branded shoes, on the grounds that they would be more 'popular'; and that they would like to wear such shoes themselves, not least for fear of being teased if they did not. Of course, asking children about brands in this way is likely to encourage them to talk about such matters at the expense of other criteria that might well be in play in real life – and in the process it runs the risk of presenting children (and poor children in particular) as 'brand slaves'. However, these children also spoke about how they had been bullied and ridiculed by their peers for wearing the 'wrong' brands, and described how they would buy such shoes partly in order to prevent this. As in Swain's (2002) study, these authors suggest that such experiences may be more common (or perhaps just more overt) among less affluent children, who are likely to experience greater pressure to want the things they cannot have.

This work is supported by a study of older children conducted by Rosaleen Croghan et al. (2006). Here again, 'style failure' – resulting from the inability to afford branded clothing – was seen as a justification for discrimination and exclusion. Children who failed to wear the correct branded clothing were marginalized, teased or harassed. Branded goods had to be genuine and purchased at full price: fakes or discounts were not permitted. Yet those who sought to win and maintain social status also had to establish their *right* to wear particular brands through other aspects of their behaviour; and for some, it felt more comfortable simply to be 'average'. Here again, the consumption and display of particular items of clothing served to establish one's legitimacy and conformity to shared norms: it served as a performance of respectability, and hence as a claim for respect (see also Phoenix, 2010). According to these authors, the style culture of the peer group is one in which economic factors (access to resources) come to be translated into ascriptions of identity and moral worth: 'style failure' becomes personal failure, the fault of the individual. Likewise, by ascribing style failure to others, we are able to distance ourselves from them, and thereby also make claims to our own moral superiority.

Similar findings appear in Tess Ridge's (2002) study of disadvantaged UK children, referred to in the previous chapter. Here again, we find instances of children making considerable efforts to disguise the evidence of their own poverty – and hence to avoid being marginalized or bullied – by strategic investments in high-status branded goods – although, as Ridge makes clear, the sense of exclusion that such children experience applies not only to aspects such as clothing but also to the ability to afford and to participate in mainstream activities among the peer group.

My account here has focused primarily on gender and social class, since it is in these areas that the most convincing research has been conducted. Some research suggests that brands can serve in a similar way as markers of ethnic identities (e.g. Bucholtz, 2007; Frosh et al., 2002; Pomerantz, 2008), albeit in ways that sometimes cut across class identifications, although – with the exception of Elizabeth Chin's (2001) work on African-American children – there has been little sustained work in this area. The relationships between brands and age identities can be seen to function in a similar way, and, as we have seen, the debate about sexualization (considered in chapter 7) can be seen at least partly as a debate about 'age-appropriateness' in children's dress.

All this work suggests that the use of clothing to signify or make claims about social identity is by no means straightforward. On the contrary, it often involves a degree of uncertainty, ambivalence and even contradiction on the part of the individual; and any claim to identity is also likely to encounter resistance from others (Pomerantz, 2008). The different parameters of social identity that I have discussed here – age, gender, social class, ethnicity – intersect in complex and sometimes unpredictable ways, and make available a wider range of (potentially competing) criteria for defining status and value: the 'rules' are never fixed, however rigid they may appear at any given time. The contemporary context of children's consumption is thus very different from the rather inflexible and static world depicted by theorists such as Pierre Bourdieu (1979): meanings have become more fluid, social hierarchies are no longer so rigid or clear-cut, and the relationships between taste and social identity have become harder to read.

Furthermore, it should be emphasized that clothing choice is also highly contingent and contextual: it does not always involve the purposeful selection, construction and display of a particular 'look', and it varies significantly in terms of what is perceived to be appropriate or suitable in a given setting (Pole et al., 2005). Particularly when it comes to children, the consumer choices that individuals make occur in the context of a network of social relationships. Parents continue to influence children's clothing choices, making judgements on the basis of moral concerns (for example, around 'sexualization') as well as economic constraints. The influence of peers may conflict with that of parents, although the peer group itself is by no means monolithic. It is also possible to overstate the emphasis on conformity in children's peer groups: as I have suggested, most young people are not members of high-status cliques, and many are content to remain merely 'average'.

On the face of it, the research presented here could be seen to lend support to popular beliefs about the harmful influence both of consumerism and of 'peer pressure', and particularly of the two acting in combination. Yet the story is more complex than this. There is no evidence here that the existence of branded goods in itself *causes* greater conflict within the peer group than would be occurring otherwise: media and consumer products may serve as a vehicle for some undesirable aspects of peer-group interaction, but they do not create them. Meanwhile, like the notion of 'pester power', the term 'peer pressure' seems to conceive of the child as a powerless victim rather than an active participant – and as somehow pathologically in thrall to the mentality of the clique. In this context, it seems to conjure up an image of 'peers' as somehow brainwashed or conscripted by marketers, marching mindlessly in lock step to the tune of the brand.

By contrast, I have argued that children actively appropriate the symbols of consumer culture in constructing their social identities and social relationships. They are not, of course, free to use them in any way they choose; and access to material goods is unequally distributed. Yet children are not dupes of the market, and they do not simply desire everything they are sold. Likewise, the peer group is by no means a singular or all-powerful force, even if many parents may perceive this to be the case (or, indeed, if children represent it in this way in making purchasing requests). On the contrary, like the family, it is itself a site of ambivalence, contradiction and resistance – as well as of meaning and pleasure. Children are not passively forced into conformity by their peers, any more than they are deluded by evil marketers into wanting things they do not really need. These latter issues lead on to a broader discussion of the role of consumption in relation to children's mental health and to 'materialism', with which this chapter concludes.

Consumption, mental health and 'materialism'

As we have seen, campaigners in this field have frequently claimed that rising commercialism has been responsible for a precipitous decline in children's mental and emotional health over recent years. This argument has been particularly prevalent in the UK in the wake of the 'toxic childhood' debate (chapter 1), and it was fuelled by a 2007 UNICEF survey that placed the UK at the bottom of an international league table of children's 'quality of life' in twenty-one industrialized countries (UNICEF, 2007). While this study looked at a range of factors, including education and material deprivation, several of the key indicators related to more subjective aspects such as the perceived quality of social relationships, 'wellbeing' and 'happiness'. However, the evidence for such claims has been widely questioned (Morrow and Mayall, 2009). Measures of 'wellbeing' are often poorly defined, and international comparisons of this kind are obviously problematic, not least because it is hard to translate key terms across languages, and because the social conventions for expressing emotions are likely to vary between cultures. Meanwhile, other studies have reported a more positive – albeit rather mixed – picture of UK childhoods (DCSF, 2007).

In terms of historical comparisons, it has been claimed that mental health problems among adolescents increased significantly between the 1970s and the late 1990s: over this period, reported problems relating to aggression and anti-social behaviour doubled, while depression increased by 50 per cent – although, perhaps surprisingly, there was no rise in Attention Deficit Hyperactivity Disorder (ADHD) (Collishaw et al., 2004). Yet the fact that more children are treated by psychiatrists and prescribed medication does not in itself indicate that mental health problems are increasing: it may merely suggest that people are more likely to report them, or indeed that such problems have been 'medicalized'. Some studies suggest that the perception of a mental health 'epidemic' is in fact due to increased levels of diagnosis (Costello et al., 2006). While some claim that these problems are caused by rising levels of affluence (O. James, 2007), others argue that they are more likely to be registered among the economically disadvantaged – which would suggest that if commercial influences do play a role here, it is likely to be a complex one.

If there is very little convincing evidence on these points, there has been rather more research on the issue of 'materialism'. However, materialism is another contested, and somewhat ill-defined, concept. Popular commentators have frequently bemoaned children's 'throwaway attitude' and their ignorance of the more meaningful things in life; and this is often accompanied by the claim that modern children are simply 'spoilt'. The accusation of 'materialism' also frequently reflects normative judgements: some material goods (most often those associated with popular culture, celebrities and fashion) are typically seen as bad, while others (particularly those associated with high culture or with education) are seen as inherently good.

Researchers have attempted to measure materialism in various ways, and numerous psychological scales have been employed. These scales are not consistent with each other, and the questions are evidently based on self-reported attitudes rather than actual behaviour. If we take materialism (in fairly crude terms) to refer to the tendency to value material things more than people, there seems to be little convincing evidence that children and young people today are becoming more materialistic than they were in earlier times. Indeed, there is a fairly extensive body of research within Political Science that suggests that the affluence of the post-war period created a generational shift in attitudes, and that young people in particular are now more inclined to espouse 'post-materialistic' values (Ingelhardt, 1981; Ingelhardt and Abramson, 1999). Social and market research surveys on these issues provide contradictory findings, and are less than reliable when it comes to making historical comparisons (e.g. Childwise, 2009; Nairn et al., 2006; Youth TGI, 2008) – although, if anything, they seem to suggest that young people regard other things as more important than the mere acquisition or possession of material goods.

Several psychological studies have suggested that individuals who hold more materialistic values tend to score lower on 'life satisfaction', perhaps because they perceive an unsatisfying gap between their current life status and some ideal to which they aspire (see Layard, 2005). Undue focus on reaching this ideal is also associated with impaired social relationships, which in turn are associated with reduced wellbeing. While there is much less evidence relating to children, the broad findings of this research are similar (e.g. Banerjee and Dittmar, 2008; Goldberg et al., 2003; Kasser et al., 2004; Schor, 2004). Particularly in their early teens, children may come to believe that buying things can solve a number of insecurity issues, such as dissatisfaction with appearance, difficulties at school, being bullied or an unhappy home life. Unpopular and insecure children feel most under pressure to conform to peer norms by buying the right brands – in effect, they seek to buy the acceptance and popularity they lack. However, questions could be raised about the validity of measures of 'life satisfaction' and 'happiness', and particularly about the difficulty of applying adult scales to children. Many of the scales used to measure wellbeing were in fact designed for medical practitioners to diagnose specific disorders such as depression, anxiety and various psychosomatic conditions.

Yet, even if the association between materialism and wellbeing in this kind of research is reasonably clear, the contribution of commercial influences is harder to assess. As we have seen, there have been studies that correlate exposure to various media with materialism (e.g. Buijzen and

Valkenburg, 2003). Children who frequently watch television commercials are more likely to express stronger materialistic values than those who do so less often, while those in lower-income families are more likely to express materialistic beliefs than those from higher-income families. However, in some cases, expected relationships between materialism, exposure to advertising and wellbeing do not appear, or are relatively weak (e.g. Nairn et al., 2010).

Here again, the key problem throughout this body of research is determining the direction of any causal relationship. It is possible that materialism causes poor wellbeing; but it is also possible that poor wellbeing leads to greater materialism, as people look to material possessions in order to cheer themselves up. Likewise, it is possible that TV viewing encourages materialistic values; but it is also possible that materialistic children watch more TV because this feeds their aspirations. Likewise, research suggests that more materialistic young people are likely to communicate more frequently with their friends, and to be more susceptible to their influence (Nairn et al., 2006). While it is possible that 'peer pressure' might foster materialism, it is equally possible that children who are more materialistic in the first place may be more inclined to communicate with friends about new purchases.

Poverty is undoubtedly a factor here, but again it seems to work in complex ways. It might seem logical that children and parents from economically deprived backgrounds would be more likely to experience commercial pressure, and hence to suffer damaging consequences, than children from more affluent backgrounds. We might then expect that pressure to be manifested, for example, in the form of higher levels of conflict within families and peer groups, lower levels of life satisfaction or self-esteem, and various other consequences in terms of physical as well as mental health. We might also expect these factors to reinforce each other, so that (for example) the unfulfilled desire for material possessions leads to reduced wellbeing, which leads in turn to a greater tendency to fantasize about such things, and hence to more materialistic attitudes.

Nevertheless, the evidence on these points is unclear. As we have seen, there is little doubt that parents in less wealthy families experience greater difficulty in dealing with their children's demands for consumer goods. However, some studies also suggest that children living in poverty may be more astute in handling money, because they have to develop the skills to do so; and that they learn to limit or adjust their demands. They also suggest that such children's consumer choices tend to favour practicality, and to be more altruistic rather than self-centred (Chin, 2001; Ridge, 2002).

Furthermore, it is by no means consistently the case that children from economically deprived backgrounds display lower levels of emotional wellbeing (see Nairn et al., 2010; Ofsted, 2007). Indeed, some studies from the US have found higher levels of depression, anxiety, substance abuse and eating disorders among children from wealthy families (e.g. Luthar, 2003; Luthar and Latendresse, 2005). This might be because such problems are more likely to be reported, although in fact it appears that wealthy parents are less likely to seek or receive help, and health professionals are less likely to sympathize with the problems of wealthy children. These researchers suggest that this higher incidence of mental health problems may arise for two reasons: parental pressure to achieve, and wealthy children's relative isolation from their parents. This research also suggests that poor people place a greater value on family togetherness, community orientation, mutual support and personal growth; and they value children for who they are, more than for what they achieve.

Conflicts with parents and peers over material goods also need to be understood in terms of family histories. For example, recent UK research suggests that the association between materialism and parent–child conflict is actually stronger for affluent children, even though 'materialism' is lower here than among poorer children (Burroughs and Rindfleisch, 2002). This may be because deprived children understand that their parents cannot afford to buy them everything they want, and are therefore less likely to be upset when their requests are refused. It may also be to do with processes of generational change, in a context of generally increasing affluence. In households where parents have experienced considerable upward mobility, the children may well expect greater material comfort than their parents enjoyed in their own childhood – yet such affluent young materialists may find their parents more interested in encouraging academic performance than in the acquisition of material goods.

Ultimately, the evidence on these issues is frustratingly limited. There may well be *associations* between poverty or inequality, higher levels of access to media, more 'materialistic' attitudes, and greater conflict within the family or the peer group; but the *causal relationships* among these factors are unclear, and in need of much further investigation.

Conclusion

In this and the previous chapter, I have explored some of the ways in which commercial factors enter into children's interpersonal relationships within the family and the peer group. However, it is hard to say whether these factors actually cause greater conflicts, or make them more likely to occur than they would otherwise do. Children are bound to argue with their parents, but there is no convincing evidence that advertising in itself (or even 'commercialism') makes this any more prevalent. Some children are unfortunately inclined to bully their peers; but if they were not doing so over clothing and footwear, they might be equally likely to focus on other aspects of physical appearance (such as weight or height or hair colour). Clearly, factors such as marketing or branding do not cause inequality, even though they may accentuate some of the more negative consequences of living with it.

People routinely use material goods to make claims about personal identity, to mediate relationships and to communicate social meanings, and, as anthropologists have shown, this is the case even in tribal or more communal societies (Douglas and Isherwood, 1979). It may well be the case, as Pugh (2009) suggests, that aspects of personal relationships such as belonging and care, as well as more negative aspects such as competitiveness and insecurity, have become 'commodified' – although this is to presume that commercial forces are somehow external to human relationships. Inequality is certainly an issue here: both parents and children may use commercial goods to signify status, and less wealthy families may struggle to avoid displaying the visible signs of poverty. Even so, this is rather different from the recurring claim that children (or indeed parents) have become more 'materialistic': if 'materialism' means anything, it is surely a symptom rather than a cause. Certainly, the research presented in these two chapters provides little support for the idea that children have come to regard objects as more important than people: if anything, it would seem that the opposite is the case.

10

Screening the market
The case of children's television

Much of the discussion in the previous chapters has focused on children's consumption of material goods (toys, food and clothing in particular), and on the impact of advertising and other promotional appeals and strategies. In this and the following chapter, the focus shifts from goods to services, in the form of broadcasting and education respectively. In the process, I also explore the ways in which broader commercial forces and pressures are determining the kinds of experiences and opportunities that are available to children.

In both of these areas, there is a long history of commercial involvement; but in the past three decades, private companies and market forces have come to play an increasingly important role. Public services have been outsourced to private companies; public sector organizations have been increasingly obliged to compete with the private sector; government regulation has been weakened or reduced; and marketized models of provision have been introduced into the delivery of public goods and services. Some of this has been apparent to the ordinary consumer, for example in the re-branding or re-badging of publicity materials; but much of it has been relatively 'invisible'. In some instances, the boundaries between public and private are now almost impossible to discern.

The involvement of commercial companies has been accompanied by other significant changes in policy and practice, to the extent that the specific effects of commercialization are difficult to identify. In some areas, most notably education, their consequences for children are likely to be long-term and extremely far-reaching – but they are not necessarily easy to establish at this point. Ultimately, however, these phenomena raise much broader questions about the kind of society we want – and, in particular, the extent to which we want a society that is largely governed by commercial imperatives.

Children's television: public service and the market

Children's television provides a particularly interesting case study of these developments. Although children's television viewing has declined somewhat in recent years, this has been by no means as dramatic as some have implied. Children have greater individualized access to a range of media technologies, but television continues to have the highest self-reported rate of consumption. This is particularly the case for younger children and for those in lower socio-economic groups. Of course, children have always spent more time watching programmes aimed at the general audience than children's programmes, although in recent years viewing in children's airtime has slightly increased as a proportion of total viewing (Ofcom, 2007c). Television – and specifically children's television – remains centrally important for children.

Historically, children have always been seen as a 'special' audience in relation to television: assumptions about their particular needs and vulnerabilities have led to the creation of specialized forms of programming, and to forms of regulation designed to protect them from material that might prove harmful. Yet, as we have seen in chapter 5, the media and cultural industries have undergone significant changes in recent years. The proliferation of media technologies and outlets, and the deregulation and globalization of markets, have had particular consequences for children's television. The question these developments pose is whether children's 'special' status can be sustained in this new environment: will all children's needs continue to be met, or will some be better served than others? The answer to this question depends largely on the extent and nature of the *value* that children are seen to represent. Are children principally seen here as a source of economic value, of profit; or are they seen to embody other symbolic, social or moral values? For what reasons, and to what extent, is it seen to be worthwhile for broadcasters to provide for children?

The history of children's television suggests that these questions have been addressed in very different ways at different times, and in different national contexts. In the following sections, I briefly trace the history of children's television in two contrasting settings: the Unites States, which has been essentially a commercial, market-led system; and the United Kingdom, which has been dominated by the ethos of public service broadcasting. Of course, in both contexts, the system of broadcasting has been rather more mixed or hybrid than this: the US has a small public sector in the form of PBS, while in the UK public service requirements – and the regulatory regime that enforces them – have always applied to terrestrial commercial broadcasters as well as to the BBC. In recent years, there have been significant changes in this respect, as the UK system has moved fairly rapidly towards a 'free-market' model – a development whose ambivalent consequences for children's television will be considered in detail later in this chapter. However, let us begin with the history.

Children in the marketplace: the US case

According to the political economist Dallas Smythe (1981), the fundamental characteristic of commercial television is that it exists in order to sell audiences to advertisers. It is the audience, not the programming, which is the commodity. The advertiser 'buys' the audience – or at least the audience's opportunity to view – while the programmes function simply as the 'bait' that entices people to watch. The more effective the broadcaster is in doing so, the more expensive the advertising rates are, and the greater are the profits. (This is not, it should be emphasized, a measure of the effectiveness of the advertising itself: what the broadcaster delivers is the availability of the audience to view, rather than guaranteeing subsequent sales.) Such a system is geared either to attracting the largest possible audience, or to delivering 'niche' audiences that are particularly desirable to advertisers (because they have higher disposable income, or prove harder to reach in other ways). Critics of such a system argue that the interests of audiences will therefore only be served insofar as they correspond to the interests of advertisers: some audience groups may be well served, while others will not.

In principle, the position of children here therefore depends primarily on how *economically* valuable they are seen to be – and this in turn depends on whether they are seen as consumers in their own right, or as a significant influence on adult consumers. If children are seen as less economically desirable than other audiences, then it makes little sense to target them specifically, and to exclude other, more valuable, audiences. We might thus expect to find schedules dominated by 'family' programming, with material that is specifically targeted at children confined to times of day when other audiences are less likely to be available to view (for example, early on Saturday mornings). Alternatively, if children are seen as more economically valuable, then we would expect to find a good deal of competition to attract them. However, this economic logic also dictates that the least possible money should be spent on programming in order to attract a given audience. If high expenditure is deemed necessary to attract especially valuable audiences, then it may be required; but if an audience of equal size and value can be retained with less expensive programming, there is little point in spending more.

Much of the history of children's television in the US appears to follow this fairly crude market logic, although economic value also interacts with what might be called *symbolic* value. The latter was particularly apparent in what William Melody (1973) calls the 'promotional era' of television in the US. While television was conceived from the very start as a commercial medium, people needed to be encouraged to invest in television sets – which in the 1950s were considerably more expensive than they are today. Children were seen to have a certain symbolic status here, at least for their parents: marketers worked hard to persuade parents that television would bring the family together, and be of benefit to children in particular, and the networks screened several hours of programmes specifically targeted at children in prime-time slots (Spigel, 1992). This has led some to regard this era as a 'Golden Age' for children's television, although there was some disparity here between the networks and the local stations, which were less interested in the children's audience and thus more likely to fill the schedules with inexpensive programmes. (There are some interesting parallels here with the early marketing of home computers, in which claims about their educational value played a key role in stimulating domestic sales: see Buckingham et al., 2001; Nixon, 1998.)

By the end of the 1950s, most families had invested in television sets, and children accordingly became a less important element of the sales pitch. Advertisers had increasingly come to exercise control, for example through sponsorship, and the emphasis was on gathering the largest possible audience. In this context, children were not considered to be of sufficient economic value, whether as consumers in their own right, or as influences on adults. Prime time was considered too precious to waste on children alone, and so children's programming was increasingly scheduled at times when other audiences were less available to view – leading to the rise of the so-called 'kid-vid ghetto' of weekend mornings. Children were generally lumped in with the family audience, which was addressed through programmes such as action-adventure shows and situation comedies that were deemed to have universal appeal (Melody, 1973; E. Palmer, 1987).

The logic of 'selling cheap' also became apparent at this time. The assumption that children would watch just about anything that they were offered led to the rise of so-called 'limited animation', notably in the form of Hanna-Barbera cartoons, which contained much less graphic detail than the cinematic work of the Disney studios, for example. Growing competition also meant that the risks of failure were higher, and hence there were few opportunities for innovation. There was a tendency to opt for repeats, spin-offs and otherwise standardized products – especially ones that could easily be sold overseas. By the end of the 1960s, over 90 per cent of children's programming on Saturday mornings was in the form of animation: there was very little live action or factual programming (Turow, 1981). There was also little attempt to cater for different groups *within* the child audience. For example, the industry believed that, while girls would watch programmes designed for boys, the opposite was not the case; and so the maxim became 'if in doubt, use boys' (Schneider, 1987).

During the 1970s, however, there was growing recognition of children as a potential market: children came to be seen as economically valuable in their own right. Advertising specifically targeted at children increased exponentially, reaching an average of 16 minutes per hour in the 'kid-vid ghetto'. While by no means new, merchandising tie-ins and commercial sponsorship of children's programmes became more widespread, with significantly greater amounts of market research addressing the children's audience. This eventually led to the emergence at the end of the decade of the so-called 'programme-length commercials', animation series produced or commissioned by toy companies as vehicles for selling their products (described in more detail in chapter 5). As we shall see in more detail later in this chapter, these developments were also further extended through the rise in specialist cable channels, which began in the mid-1980s in the US: with the mass audience in decline, children came to be regarded as a 'demographically pure' audience, and hence as a significant 'niche' market.

The increasing commercial targeting of children was made possible – and indeed actively encouraged – by the general climate of deregulation. However, it did not go uncontested. Citizen activism – most notably in the form of the organization Action for Children's Television (ACT) – grew significantly during the 1970s; and while its targets were often quite broad-ranging, there was a key focus on the dominance of advertising. ACT mobilized protectionist arguments about children's vulnerability to advertising, sometimes in rather crude ways (see Hendershot, 1998; Seiter, 1993), but it also focused on the broader implications of a commercially dominated system in terms of scheduling, the diversity and quality of programming, and the attention to children's needs. In the short term, ACT's efforts in lobbying the Federal Communications Commission (FCC: the leading regulatory body in the US) made relatively little headway; and they were significantly knocked back by the adoption of a more vigorously 'free-market' stance under the Reagan government of the 1980s. In the words of Dale Kunkel (1988), the FCC's stance at this time changed 'from a raised eyebrow to a turned back': many regulatory constraints on advertising were swept away, and positive requirements for the provision of children's programming were removed. However, in the early 1990s, under a Democratic administration, the tide turned somewhat: the Children's Television Act of 1990 stipulated requirements for stations to provide 'educational' programmes – and while these were initially interpreted in a very loose manner, the regulations were subsequently tightened in 1996. Even so, regulation in this sector remains comparatively weak: generally speaking, it is largely reactive, in response to public complaints, rather than proactive.

To sum up this brief history, broadcasting in the US is essentially a competitive, commercial system, with relatively little government regulation. This kind of arrangement is, of course, one that is frequently justified by free-market economists as the most efficient way of meeting consumers' needs: the market, they argue, will provide. Equally, it is often condemned by critics as a system that is fundamentally incapable of meeting needs: the market, as Kline (1993) and others suggest, will *never* provide (see chapter 3). However, this partly depends upon how those 'needs' are conceived of in the first place. Historically, the extent to which children's needs – in terms of the quantity, diversity and quality of television programming – have been met has depended very significantly on the varying ways in which the economic, symbolic and social *value* of children has been understood.

Childhood and public service: the UK case

The history of the television system in the UK has been quite different, for a variety of reasons. Compared with the US, there is generally a very different view of the relationships between commerce and government, and a stronger tradition of public welfare provision, while, in terms of television, there have until recently been many fewer channels, and a much more centralized national system. As we shall see, these differences have significant implications for children's television in particular.

The history of public service broadcasting in the UK has been told countless times, and there is little point in rehearsing it here (concise accounts can be found in Crisell, 2002; and Curran and Seaton, 2009). Lord John Reith, the founder of the BBC, famously saw broadcasting as a kind of cultural mission: it would bring about the 'cultural uplift' of the general population, and serve as a powerful means of securing a strong national identity. Critical discussions of public service broadcasting have frequently made much of Reith's undeniable paternalism, but there are some fundamental principles here that can be defined in more neutral terms (e.g. Murdock, 1990). Public service broadcasting is required through legislation to offer a balance of 'information, education and entertainment'; to be universally available to all; to cater for specific minority audiences (including children); and to provide quality and diversity in programming. In the revised definition recently proposed by the regulator Ofcom (2007c), it also has a responsibility to stimulate interest and knowledge in areas such as science, the humanities and the arts, and to reflect and strengthen cultural identity and cultural awareness.

Public service broadcasting should not be confused with public *sector* broadcasting – that is, the BBC. The BBC is funded not through advertising or commercial sponsorship, but by a form of compulsory taxation (the licence fee). Since 1955, the BBC has sat alongside terrestrial commercial broadcasters, which carry advertising. However, these companies are also regulated and monitored in order to ensure that they follow public service principles. Some have argued that this mixed (public/commercial) system has historically helped to temper the BBC's tendency towards paternalism, while the strength of the BBC has helped to keep the commercial companies 'honest'. (It should be noted here that these public service requirements do not apply to cable and satellite broadcasters.)

Under the British public service system, children have historically been defined as a special audience, with particular needs and vulnerabilities that differ from those of adults. This special status has been manifested in a range of ways. In terms of scheduling, for example, broadcasters have been required to provide programmes in specified slots at times when children are most likely to be able to view (such as late afternoons), irrespective of whether other, more commercially valuable, audiences (such as 'housewives') are also available. In terms of diversity, broadcasters have been required to provide information, education and entertainment; to offer a range of programme genres, including factual programmes and live action drama as well as animation and entertainment; and to cater for different needs across the full age range. Quality is a more debatable issue, of course; but historically broadcasters have been required to invest in forms of programming at a level that is not necessarily justified (in the case of commercial channels) by the return from advertising. For example, this means that children's programmes must include relatively costly forms such as live action drama, as well as programmes that are culturally specific to the UK and that might be difficult or impossible to sell in overseas markets.

If these are the broad principles, there have been some significant historical changes in terms of how they are realized in relation to children. Our research (Buckingham et al., 1999) showed that definitions of childhood and understandings of children's 'needs' and 'wants' have been the subject of constant, unresolved debate among television professionals. While the BBC Children's Department originally enjoyed a monopoly, its position was seriously unsettled by the successful emergence of commercial television (ITV) in the late 1950s. BBC producers and policy-makers struggled to understand the cultural meaning and practical implications of children's preference for the entertainment-oriented output of ITV, above the more worthy, but rather staid, programming of the BBC (see also Oswell, 2002; and Wagg, 1992). On the one hand, the BBC felt bound to defend a notion of childhood which it acknowledged was both nation-centred and constructed around 'middle-class' norms of behaviour; while, on the other, it had to recognize majority preferences for 'commercial' American-influenced programmes, often in genres – cartoons, for example – which affronted more conservative tastes. Ultimately, this was a debate that could not be resolved within the existing regime. After a period of internal crisis, the BBC's Children's Department was closed down in the early 1960s: it was subsumed by a new Family Department, and when it re-emerged later in the decade, it did so with a much less paternalistic view of its audience.

In the 1970s, the public service ethos was further modernized, as the BBC began to engage with a wider range of children's cultures: there was growing recognition of pop music, for example; a new emphasis on children's autonomy and independent 'voice'; and increasing representation of aspects of working-class children's experience. However, these developments were accompanied by persistent arguments about 'Americanization' and the necessity for children's television to reflect national cultures and patterns of social life. Even so, this period of the 'regulated duopoly', in which the BBC and ITV were the sole providers, was one of considerable stability: while the commercial channel did provoke innovation, it was also subject to regulation (through a series of interventions from the Pilkington Report of 1962 to the Broadcasting Act of 1990) that required consistent levels of investment and provision for children.

In the 1980s and 1990s, multi-sided market competition, involving globalized media corporations, became an increasingly important feature of the landscape of children's broadcasting in the UK. In the late 1990s, there was a proliferation of specialist cable/satellite channels for children; and while the generic range of new programming was comparatively narrow, much of it appeared distinctly fresh and innovative, and there was a great deal more for children to choose from. Like the BBC in the 1950s, the established terrestrial broadcasters struggled to come to terms with new competition. While its audience has been somewhat eroded, the BBC's children's programming has since continued to enjoy relatively high levels of funding, although it has also come to depend upon co-production, merchandising and global sales. By contrast, as we shall see below, children's programming on the main commercial terrestrial channel (ITV1) is now in steep decline.

These economic and institutional changes have been reflected in changing conceptions of the child audience. Our interviews with television producers, conducted in the late 1990s, identified four overlapping definitions or discourses about the child audience (Buckingham et al., 1999). The first centres on the idea of the *vulnerable* child – the child who is threatened by the bad effects of television or at risk of being seduced by consumer culture, and for both reasons is seen to be in need of protection. The second is a *'child-centred'* discourse, in which ideas about children's essential nature, the stages of their development and their consequent needs are used to justify particular kinds of scheduling and programme-making. The third and fourth types of discourse assume that children are articulate social actors, rather than merely in development ('beings' rather than 'becomings': see chapter 3). They are similar in that they stress the primacy of children's preferences and draw attention to children's social capabilities. They differ in that they inflect the socially active child in conceptually distinct – though overlapping – ways: the child is variously understood either as a *consumer* or as a potential *citizen*. Of course, these ideas themselves reflect changing conceptions of childhood more broadly; and they can also be seen as responses to economic changes both in broadcasting and in consumer culture.

At first glance, the story of post-war broadcasting in the UK suggests a chronological development of these models, although in contemporary discussions of children's television, all these discourses – which developed at different historical moments – are in fact simultaneously present. Nevertheless, they are not equal in status. Protectionism still has considerable influence as a public discourse about television, but as an occupational ideology among professionals it has a less commanding position. Child-centredness remains important but has lost the secure institutional basis on which it once flourished, and depends for its survival on a fraught and unceasing negotiation with the pressures of the marketplace. The third discourse – the model of the child as active consumer – is increasingly prominent, and is the favoured language of cable/satellite producers. Finally, the second strand of the 'child as social actor' discourse – one that focuses on children as citizens – influences minority programming and has a special public status in the corporate declarations of media professionals.

Despite these changes and ongoing conflicts, it is clear that UK public service broadcasting has historically rested on a very different conception of the *value* of the child audience from the one that is embodied in the US commercial system. To be sure, in the UK the child does have a certain *symbolic* value for parents; and when seeking to defend the licence fee, the BBC tends to resort to very traditional representations of childhood innocence that it imagines will appeal to parents' 'better nature' (Buckingham, 2002b). However, there is also a broader conception of children's needs here that is not primarily to do with their economic value as consumers. Rather, there is a sense of responsibility towards children themselves that is fundamentally *ethical* in nature (Oswell, 2002). It is important to emphasize that this is not something that is primarily defined in terms of *education* – as it is, for example, in the US Children's Television Act. Indeed, UK children's television producers have always been quite resistant to the idea that the purpose of their work should be seen primarily in educational terms: children's television can be *educative*, but it should not be narrowly *educational*. Rather, children are seen to be entitled to television as a form of public good – and indeed as a necessary *cultural* experience.

Children's television in the noughties

The picture I have outlined thus far has offered a contrast between two 'ideal types' – and, as such, it is perhaps unduly schematic. Nevertheless, much of the public debate about children's television in the UK tends to represent the situation in even more stark and binary terms. According to some campaigners, the 'great tradition' of public service broadcasting is now in terminal decline, as British children's screens have come to be dominated by a flood of cheap US imports (Blumler, 1992; Blumler and Bilfereyst, 1998; and see Buckingham et al., 1999). Children's television, they argue, is being 'dumbed down', standards of quality are being eroded, and fundamental values to do with citizenship and children's social development are being abandoned in favour of pleasing advertisers. Unless something is done now, British children will apparently be consigned to a future of wall-to-wall American cartoons.

This kind of argument rests on a series of oppositions and assumptions that are highly problematic. The British public service tradition is equated with quality and responsibility, while the US system is typically seen as a purveyor of worthless junk. While public service television is about doing children good, commercial television is about exploiting them; while public service gives children what they need, commercial television simply gives them what they want. These polarities – at least in the discourse of some campaigners – seem to rest on some unstated assumptions about cultural value: cartoons, for example, are typically seen as inherently bad, while live action drama (preferably based on literary adaptations) is inherently good; entertainment is seen as inherently bad, while education is bound to be good; commercial television is incapable of delivering 'quality', while public service effectively guarantees it. In the British context, this argument also rests on assumptions about national identity. Campaigners who are concerned about the rise in imported programmes frequently claim that British children *should* see images of British life on screen – although this tends to presume that 'Britishness' is a singular and coherent identity, and avoids the question of *whose* 'British' lives are to be represented (for further discussion, see Buckingham et al., 1999).

Yet if these polarities are problematic in themselves, they also bear little relationship to contemporary realities. While the system in the UK has been driven by a strong public service ethos, it has always entailed a dynamic relationship between the public and the private sector. The UK has always had a 'mixed economy' in broadcasting – albeit a regulated one, of a particular historical kind. There are certainly some ways in which the operation of the market makes broadcasting more accountable or responsive to popular tastes and needs than public broadcasting, although there other ways in which the market cannot – or at least does not – provide. Yet in the current context, the distinction between the two has become increasingly blurred; and the consequences of this for children are complex and ambivalent. Before moving on to consider the likely future of children's television, this section discusses two contrasting instances that illustrate some of the broader forces that are currently in play: namely, the BBC and the specialist children's channel Nickelodeon.[1]

The BBC

In recent years, the BBC has undergone a significant shift in the direction of both commercialization and marketization. It has been increasingly forced to compete with its commercial rivals, and to generate revenue both from merchandising and other 'spin-offs', and from international co-productions and overseas sales. It has also been internally 'marketized', or reorganized along market lines: it is required to outsource a certain quota of its programming, and departments are obliged to compete and to finance their activities in a form of internal market (see Born, 2004). Meanwhile, its legitimacy has increasingly been called into question; and as its audience share inevitably declines, it is under growing pressure to justify the licence fee and to display public accountability. It has moved quite aggressively into cable / satellite broadcasting, and developed its online activities, although here it is vulnerable to the charge that these services are not available to all licence fee payers.

These competing economic and cultural imperatives have been particularly apparent in its children's programming. Children carry a considerable economic value here, as a source of income from ancillary goods and services, and from international programme sales. Thus, for example, the BBC has developed two specialist cable / satellite channels, as well as a growing range of children's websites and online services; and it has generated increasing revenue from in-house publications and products, as well as licensed toys and other merchandise. Yet, at the same time, children are seen to carry a considerable symbolic value. For campaigners, children's television has been regarded as a kind of litmus test of public service, and the BBC has been keen to proclaim its continuing sense of ethical responsibility here.

To date, the BBC has managed to resolve these competing imperatives most successfully in relation to the pre-school market – which, as I have noted, appears to have grown significantly in recent years (see chapter 5). Jeanette Steemers (2010) provides a detailed analysis of the broader 'ecology' of contemporary pre-school television in the UK, which draws attention to some of the tensions between commercial and public service imperatives. As she argues, the proliferation of new channels has led to an increasing fragmentation of audiences, and this has encouraged broadcasters to develop distinct brands for different sub-sections of the child audience. However, they are also increasingly dependent upon co-financing, international sales and ancillary merchandise in order to finance production – although 'big hits' in merchandising are comparatively rare.

Partly building on its public service heritage, the BBC is an exceptionally powerful brand in this market, both in the UK and globally; and its specialist channel for this age group, CBeebies, has been particularly successful. CBeebies is a 'tri-media' brand, available on cable / satellite and terrestrial television (BBC2), as well as radio and online. The emphasis here is very much on the potential of learning through play, addressing children's developmental needs, and building confidence and a sense of community. However, the BBC has not always managed to maintain the distinction between *educational* and *educative* programming here; and some of the ancillary publications (magazines and software) that have emerged from its pre-school programming adopt a highly didactic approach, perhaps in order to appeal to conventional ideas about what counts as 'good' education (Buckingham and Scanlon, 2003). Meanwhile, such programming is also a powerful means of generating revenue, both through international sales and through merchandise: children's content currently generates just under £70 million annually for the BBC's commercial arm, BBC Worldwide (Steemers, 2010).

Some of the tensions at stake here were apparent in the case of *Teletubbies*, without doubt one of the most successful and influential children's programmes of recent years. Since its launch in 1997, the programme has been sold in more than sixty countries worldwide, and translated into over forty languages. Millions of pounds have been generated from *Teletubbies* videos, magazines, computer games, toys and other merchandise. *Teletubbies* is an outsourced, independent production, although much of the commercial activity surrounding it has been licensed through BBC Worldwide. It is clear that an investment of this scale (260 programmes were originally commissioned) could not have been sustained without the possibility of such funding being identified at an early stage. Yet while the programme rapidly became popular with the child audience, it also attracted widespread critical condemnation: it was accused of abandoning the 'great tradition' of educative programming, and thereby 'dumbing down' its audience; and of commercially exploiting young children. The BBC's sensitivity to such accusations can be seen as a symptomatic reflection of its current dilemmas, as it attempts to sustain national public service traditions while simultaneously depending on commercial activities and global sales. (For further discussion, see Buckingham, 2002a.)

Nickelodeon

Nickelodeon has been one of the most striking success stories of commercial children's broadcasting. Launched in the late 1970s, and now owned by the US media giant Viacom, it also has significant interests in online media, movies, print publications, character toys, theme parks and other merchandising. Nickelodeon is a global brand, which is apparently now available in 100 million households worldwide – although it should be noted that most of its programming is US-made, and it invests comparatively little in local production. While the Nickelodeon channel was originally aimed at children more broadly, the company has since launched a specialist pre-school channel, Nick Jr., while in the US there is a further spin-off in the form of Nicktoons, devoted solely to animation. Programming on the main Nickelodeon channel is dominated by animation; and it is fair to say that it has created some of the most innovative examples of this genre in recent years, from *Rugrats* and *Ren and Stimpy* to *Spongebob Squarepants*. However, it has also included sitcoms and variety shows, and one of the few news magazine programmes for children, *Nick News* (see Buckingham, 2000b), while the programmes on Nick Jr. include live-action shows such as *Blue's Clues* alongside 'educational' animations such as *Dora the Explorer*.

Like the BBC, Nickelodeon has sought in various ways to combine commercial and public service imperatives – although there is no regulatory requirement, either in the UK or the US, for it to address the latter. Nevertheless, the rhetoric and branding of Nickelodeon is strikingly different from that of the BBC. Certainly, in addressing parents, the BBC still tends to hark back to the past, invoking (or indeed re-inventing) tradition – and, in the process, playing to parents' nostalgia for the television of their own childhoods. By contrast, Nickelodeon does not have to achieve legitimacy with parents (and hence secure their continued assent for the compulsory licence fee): it can address children directly, and it does so in ways that emphasize their 'wacky' anarchic humour and their sensuality (see Buckingham, 2002b).

Nevertheless, there are clearly some tensions here. On the one hand, Nickelodeon's executives are keen to emphasize the pro-social, broadly educational dimensions of its work, and to reassure parents that the channel is a non-violent 'safe space' for children (e.g. H. Jenkins, 2004; Laybourne, 1993). Thus, the channel quite frequently runs campaigns and events relating to issues such as volunteering, the environment and healthy eating; and Nick Jr. in particular is 'sold' on the basis of its educational credentials. Yet, on the other hand, the main Nickelodeon channel also adopts a rhetoric of empowerment – a notion of the channel as giving voice to kids, taking the kids' point of view, as the friend of kids. This is frequently aligned with a form of 'anti-adultism', which defines adults as necessarily boring and conservative (Banet-Weiser, 2004; Simensky, 2004) – although, as Heather Hendershot (2004) has noted, this apparent subversiveness in itself also has a significant 'transgenerational' appeal.

However, this discourse also places a strong emphasis on children's active participation: children are urged to become 'agents of change', and to engage in forms of civic action in their communities. This rhetoric could be seen as a symptomatic instance of the ways in which market values have come to be aligned with liberal political discourses about children's rights (as discussed in chapter 5). As Sarah Banet-Weiser (2007) suggests, it could be seen to represent a new form of 'consumer-citizenship', which combines purchasing power with an assertion of children's growing social and even political power. From this perspective, the channel's emphasis on particular notions of 'girl power' or 'diversity' would be seen not just as politically correct window-dressing but rather as grounds for a new kind of enfranchisement of children – albeit within the terms of consumer culture.

Interestingly, the differences between the BBC and Nickelodeon are significantly more apparent on the older children's channels than on the pre-school channels (Bailey, 2010). The pedagogical style of Nick Jr. has much in common with that of CBeebies: there is a shared emphasis on 'child-centred' values of care, nurture and play – although, if anything, Nick Jr. tends to espouse a more didactic approach. By contrast, the main Nickelodeon channel is significantly more wild and anarchic in style than its BBC equivalent, CBBC; while the latter is more informed by notions of responsibility and social development, Nickelodeon presents itself primarily in terms of humour and fun, and as the antithesis of school and of adulthood.

The comparison between the BBC and Nickelodeon suggests that any easy opposition between public service and commercial systems is misleading, and no longer corresponds to contemporary realities. While there are certainly differences in the kinds of programmes and services they provide, and in the broader ethos of the channels, these are by no means absolute. Indeed, in practice there is considerable synergy between them. There have been several instances of co-productions, while the BBC currently screens some Nickelodeon shows in the UK, and vice versa. The notion that public service broadcasting is somehow exclusively able to meet children's needs or to guarantee 'quality' is one that cannot be sustained. However, this is not in any way to suggest that the distinction is no longer meaningful – as might be implied by Nickelodeon's company slogan, 'what's good for kids is good for business'. The more difficult challenge for future policy is to identify precisely where and in what ways the market will *not* provide.

Children's television in crisis?

As I have suggested, the boundaries between the public and the private in British children's broadcasting have become extremely blurred in recent years. UK terrestrial broadcasters now face intensifying competition, both from cable and satellite providers and from other digital media; their budgets are squeezed, and they are required to earn increasing amounts of their revenue from merchandising and global sales; government regulation has come to exercise a significantly lighter touch; traditional advertising is in decline, and income now has to be generated across multiple media platforms; and the BBC in particular has faced growing criticisms of its apparently privileged position. Over the past twenty years, a succession of reports – many of them produced by regulatory bodies such as the former Broadcasting Standards Commission and (most recently) by Ofcom – has suggested that children's television may be 'in crisis' – although it remains to be seen whether this is merely a matter of temporary adjustment or a more fundamental, long-term problem (Blumler, 1992; Cowling and Lee, 2002; M. Davies and Corbett, 1997). In fact, the implications of these developments for children would seem to be quite ambivalent. Ofcom's report *The Future of Children's Television Programming* (2007c), on which the following paragraphs draw, provides some interesting findings in this respect.

On one level, it is clear that the sheer quantity of children's television available – at least to the majority of UK families that subscribe to cable or satellite – has vastly increased, multiplying approximately six-fold over the past ten years. However, the provision on terrestrial channels has remained relatively constant, and has recently fallen slightly, most notably on the commercial terrestrial channels ITV1 and Channel 4. The overall increase in airtime has inevitably resulted in a considerable rise in the proportion of repeats. More importantly, most of the new material is US in origin; most of it is closely integrated with toys and other merchandise based on licensed characters; and most of it is confined to a narrow range of genres – primarily cartoon animation and situation comedy. There has been a marked decline in the provision of UK-originated programmes commissioned by the commercial terrestrial broadcasters, whose expenditure on first-run original content halved between 1998 and 2006.

Meanwhile, the advent of new technologies, combined with the growing interest in the children's market, has led to a phenomenal proliferation of specialist children's channels, of which there are currently almost thirty in the UK. As I have noted, the BBC has enjoyed considerable success with its two dedicated channels, especially CBeebies, while ITV has entered this market more recently. However, all the other channels are owned by major US-based companies, notably Disney, Turner and Viacom; and most are only available via subscription packages. These channels devote very little funding to the production of original UK-sourced material (around 10 per cent of total investment in new programming), and their UK productions are largely produced with an eye to global sales. While these new channels have very small audience shares, they have grown as children have begun to migrate from the terrestrial broadcasters. At the same time, while households with children are more likely to have cable/satellite (which of course have to be paid for through subscription), there are still around 10 per cent that do not.

Children's television has always been a relatively 'protected' area on terrestrial commercial channels in the UK, in the sense that more is spent on it than is retrieved in advertising revenue. However, the recent rise in the quantity of children's programming has been accompanied by a general decline in advertising and subscription revenue, making children's television even less commercially attractive. The high degree of competition between channels and the fragmentation of the audience inevitably drives down the value of each channel for advertisers. Meanwhile, buying-in programmes is almost invariably cheaper than original production, because of the economies of scale in the global market, and so the increasing amounts of schedule time available are likely to become ever more dominated by imported programmes and by repeats. With declining income from broadcasters, producers are also becoming correspondingly more reliant on income from ancillary merchandise and sales in global markets.

Meanwhile, there have been some significant changes in the regulatory regime affecting children's television. The 2003 Communications Act brought in a more flexible self-regulatory (or co-regulatory) approach. Among other things, it removed the requirement for mandated levels or quotas of children's programming on these channels. As such, broadcasters are now able to decide the amount and the nature of what they deliver in this area, although Ofcom is able to consider whether such channels include a 'suitable quantity and range of high-quality and original programmes for children and young people'. This was followed by the introduction of the new regulations relating to HFSS food advertising, which broadcasters argued was bound to lead to a fall in advertising revenue (see chapter 6). In 2008, Ofcom allowed ITV1, the leading terrestrial commercial channel, to reduce its hours for children's programmes, effectively ending the protected late afternoon slot (Steemers, 2010).

The most dramatic consequence of these developments has been the reduction in investment in original programming among the terrestrial commercial broadcasters. ITV1, in particular, has now effectively abandoned its funding of UK children's programmes. Although it was argued that this was in response to a decline in income following the new HFSS regulations, it has in fact been the latest step in a long-term shift over the past decade. This leaves the BBC in an exposed position, as by far the leading investor in UK-produced programmes, particularly factual programmes and drama; and questions are being raised about the need for a plurality of providers. Although it currently offers more children's programming than is required by its service licences, the BBC could in theory reduce its output quite significantly.

All these changes impact in different ways on different genres of programming. Broadly speaking, animation and pre-school programmes are much easier to sell in global markets than live action drama or factual programmes. The more culturally specific a drama programme is, the less likely it is to sell – although there are some exceptions to this. Programmes with significant merchandising or other 'spin-off' possibilities (for example in the form of computer games or educational software) are more lucrative than those with limited potential of this kind. Programmes with a longer 'shelf life', which do not date so quickly, such as pre-school programmes and animation, are also more attractive investments – for example, as compared with factual programmes. In addition, some genres of programming (most notably live action drama) are generally more expensive to produce than others. This has resulted in a situation where companies are reluctant to invest, for example, in contemporary non-comedy drama; and this in turn accentuates the tendency to marginalize programmes that reflect specifically British cultural experiences and values.

Ofcom's report (2007c) also draws attention to some important differences in the implications here for different age groups. In general, it finds that pre-school and younger children are well served by existing programming, but that older children (aged 9–12) and especially young teenagers are more poorly served, especially in respect of original UK drama and factual programmes. Ofcom's research also suggests that parents are relatively dissatisfied, particularly with the output of commercial terrestrial channels – although the BBC, including its dedicated channels, fares significantly better. Parents of pre-school and younger children are generally more satisfied, although parents of older children, and older children themselves, feel they are less well served, particularly in respect of drama and factual programmes that specifically target their age group.

In broad terms, then, the changing nature of children's programming in the UK is coming to reflect the 'market logic' identified earlier in this chapter. This is most evident on the terrestrial commercial channels. If various potential audiences are available to view, the most lucrative audience (in terms of advertising revenue) is more likely to be targeted; and companies are also likely to take the least expensive means to reach a given audience. In this context, effects may also become causes. Thus, if teenagers find that there are relatively few programmes specifically addressing them, they may come to prefer other screen media to television; and in this context, broadcasters may then feel there is little point in providing dedicated programming for them, particularly if they can be reached through mainstream adult output.

As such, the future prospects for children's television appear quite uncertain. Some sectors of the children's market – notably pre-schoolers, and to some extent younger children – are being better served in terms of the quantity, as well as (more arguably) the range and quality, of programming, although others are rather worse off than before. Some UK companies, including the BBC, are major players in the global children's television market; and some US-owned cable/satellite channels also recognize the 'brand value' of UK-originated production. Even so, it is hard to see how the UK children's market can sustain the current level of competition – and especially the ever-growing number of dedicated channels. Another possibility here is that the internet will come to fill the place once occupied by children's television, although the potential here is limited. While the BBC's websites are popular with children, they are funded from the licence fee and from income deriving from ancillary merchandise. Beyond this, the internet remains a largely unregulated commercial medium, and there is no clearly sustainable model for funding public service content for children online.

Yet a further question here is whether any of this matters to children themselves. What would be the impact on children if UK-produced children's television effectively disappeared, and if the only programmes available were animation series delivered by the US-owned cable/satellite companies? In debating these issues, campaigners are almost bound to appeal to arguments about cultural and educational values. For instance, they argue that British children *should* see representations of British children on their television screens, and that this plays a significant role in the formation of national cultural identity and citizenship. Likewise, they argue that children *should* see a range of different types of programming designed for their age group – including live action drama, news and documentary, rather than merely animation; and they suggest that this is essential for their socialization and healthy cultural development. These arguments may well be persuasive, but there is little research that would support them: they are normative judgements rather than ones that can be proven by appealing to evidence.

Conclusion

The example of children's television provides a particularly interesting case study of the implications of the shift towards a more commercialized media environment. However, the implications of this shift for children themselves are far from clear. There is some evidence that children from less affluent families who do not have access to subscription channels are likely to be worse off, as the provision on terrestrial television is reduced; and such children are also less likely to have access to alternatives such as broadband internet. Nevertheless, the market has made available a significantly increased amount of programming specifically targeted at children. Of course, quantity is not the same as quality or diversity, but the picture here is by no means straightforward. There are some grounds for suggesting that the range of programming available to children has narrowed, but quality is much more difficult to ascertain. In certain areas – most notably animation and pre-school, but also some forms of 'participatory' programming – commercial providers have been a significant force for innovation. Even if the *public sector* of television is now a much smaller part of the broader landscape, there is rather less convincing evidence that *public service values* have been entirely abandoned. As in the case of Nickelodeon's 'consumer citizenship', it is possible that we are seeing new hybrid forms emerging – although the extent to which these are being taken up by children themselves is an issue that is in need of further research and debate.

11

Consuming to learn – learning to consume

Education goes to market

Schooling – and education more broadly – is an increasingly important arena for children's encounters with consumer culture. Many key aspects of what was formerly public educational provision – from school buildings and facilities to teacher training and examinations – are now provided and run by private companies. Commercial businesses provide an extensive range of teaching materials for use in the classroom, as well as sponsoring school programmes and initiatives, providing 'free' equipment, and using schools as venues for advertising and market research. Alongside formal schooling, companies are also offering supplementary classes and private tutoring, as well as marketing a growing selection of educational books, magazines, CD-ROMs and websites for use in the home. Although many of these are by no means new phenomena, they have all significantly increased in scale over the past two decades.

This chapter focuses on five main aspects of this phenomenon. In respect of schools, I consider three distinct but related processes: commercialization – that is, the presence of advertising messages and marketing activities in schools; privatization – that is, the provision by private companies of educational services that were formerly provided by the public sector; and marketization – that is, the reorganization of public education according to market principles. I then move on to consider two aspects of learning outside schools: the commercial marketing of educational goods and services; and the commercialization of children's leisure and play. As I shall attempt to show, these are complementary developments, which are all contributing to broader shifts in the nature and meaning of learning in contemporary consumer societies.

Ultimately, it may be unrealistic – or even utopian – to expect that schools should be entirely insulated from the operations of the market economy. However, as in the case of children's broadcasting, there are significant ethical and political questions here about the extent to which public services should be governed by commercial imperatives, and about the consequences of this for children. This in turn raises questions about how schools and teachers might respond to such developments, and about what children need to learn about the operations of the market. These questions will be addressed in the concluding sections of this chapter.

A history of ambivalence

As we have seen, children are often described as a particularly volatile market, which is becoming harder for marketers to understand and to reach. In this context, schools have often been seen as a valuable arena for advertising and marketing. As long ago as the 1920s, schools in the United States were being supplied with commercially branded 'enrichment materials' in the form of booklets, wallcharts and films. School books were adorned with advertising, corporate salesmen and entertainers were invited into schools, and children were given vouchers and invited to participate in competitions that would encourage their parents to add particular products to their shopping lists (Jacobson, 2004). Such activities attracted criticism – in 1929, the US National Education Association published a report warning teachers about the dangers of 'free' corporate handouts – but they appear to have been welcomed by many teachers. By the end of the 1970s, a report for Ralph Nader's Centre for the Study of Responsive Law entitled *Hucksters in the Classroom* (Harty, 1979) found that commercially sponsored teaching materials were very widely used in schools, and often contained misleading forms of 'industry propaganda'.

However, such overt forms of marketing are only part of a bigger picture. As Larry Cuban (2004) shows, the involvement of business in schools has a broader history, at least in the United States, which runs from the vocational education initiatives of the early twentieth century through to the target-driven, privatized education markets of the past decade. The incursion of business interests in public education – for example in the form of corporate sponsorship, employment training programmes, and for-profit schools – has been accompanied by a range of reforms designed to make schools more 'business-like' in their operation and governance.

Such activities are often legitimated through a rhetoric of 'partnership', through which schools receive funding in cash or in kind in return for providing companies with access to children. Companies frequently present their involvement with schools as a form of altruism or social responsibility, a matter of 'giving something back', and are often less than transparent about the return on investment it provides in terms of promoting their brands. Nevertheless, this relationship has always been a somewhat ambivalent one. In Cuban's account, such activities form part of a broader history of attempts at top-down reform that have largely ignored the working conditions of schools and denigrated the professional expertise of teachers. Cuban argues that many of these initiatives have failed because they have neglected the fundamental – and indeed necessary – differences between businesses and schools. Children and parents, he argues, are not merely 'customers': schools have to serve broader social purposes in respect of citizenship, and be accountable to the public in doing so. As this implies, there may be an inevitable tension here between the public mission of the school and the private interests of business.

Commercialization: marketing in schools

The most visible aspects of this phenomenon relate to commercialization – that is, the presence of commercial marketing and advertising in schools. Alex Molnar, who has conducted regular annual reviews of commercial involvement in US schools over many years (see, for example, Molnar, 2005; Molnar and Boninger, 2007), provides a useful typology of the different forms this takes. This includes the following:

- sponsorship, for example of school events and activities;
- exclusive agreements with companies for the provision of goods and services (typically in exchange for a share of profits);
- incentive programmes, such as voucher or token schemes;
- appropriation of school space for logos, banners or advertising hoardings;
- sponsored or branded teaching materials or lesson plans;
- electronic marketing (the provision of television or computer equipment or services for schools in exchange for the right to advertise);
- commercial programmes or packages designed to assist schools with fundraising.

Further categories here might include:

- the use of schools as venues for market research on students;
- sponsored equipment (particularly computer equipment);
- marketing events or programmes, such as commercial book clubs;
- awards, prizes or 'kitemarks' offered by companies for achievement in particular areas;
- distribution of free samples.

As Jane Kenway and Elizabeth Bullen (2001) point out, such activities have several apparent benefits for companies. They enable them to target specific 'niches' among the broader children's market, to build brand loyalty from an early age, and to establish a philanthropic image (not least for the benefit of parents). In a context of declining interest in television advertising, and stricter regulation in some areas, they provide an alternative form of marketing that can be much less overt. The apparent benefits for schools are even more self-evident; and as critics suggest, such practices have proven particularly attractive to less well-funded schools in poorer neighbourhoods, especially in the United States, where there are significant inequalities in school funding (Linn, 2004). Although reliable statistics would probably be difficult to obtain (Molnar's research looks only at press reports), it seems fair to conclude that these activities have grown significantly in scope and scale in recent years.

According to Molnar and Boninger (2007), commercial involvement in US schools has gradually shifted away from 'hard sell' advertising towards a more subtle, and more pervasive, approach. For example, Channel One – a service in which schools are provided with 'free' television receiving equipment in exchange for the compulsory daily screening of a news programme containing advertising – seems now to be in decline, although at one point it was claiming to serve 40 per cent of US middle and high schools (see De Vaney, 1994). A similar service called Bus Radio, which plays music with commercials on school buses, is still growing, although (like Channel One) it has attracted widespread criticism.[1] However, Molnar argues that companies are now moving towards a much less direct approach, based on branding and 'customer relationship management' rather than advertising per se. This is in line with the more general shift in marketing strategies (described in chapter 5) towards a more 'participatory' approach. Marketers recognize that in this context more overt forms of marketing are also more likely to attract public criticism, and hence may prove counter-productive in terms of cultivating a positive brand image (Siegel et al., 2001). As Kenway and Bullen (2001) show, companies pay careful attention to the 'ethical management' of such activities, seeking to cultivate long-term partnerships, and to infuse commercial messages with pro-social, morale-boosting or 'politically correct' content.

Marketing and advertising in UK schools

While some of these forms of commercial involvement are much further developed (and much less regulated) in the US, most exist in some form in the UK as well. Some are well known, such as the national 'Computers for Schools' voucher programme offered by the supermarket Tesco, but others are smaller-scale and less obviously visible. Examples of leading companies involved include Nestlé, McDonalds and Unilever, although, on a smaller scale, many local businesses also sponsor school events or activities. A whole range of companies – from financial services and energy companies through to Google and Disney – provide teaching materials for schools, and there are numerous advertising-supported sites offering 'free' classroom resources. As might be expected in light of growing concerns about obesity (see chapter 6), food and drink companies are especially prominent here, for example in providing resources and facilities, sponsoring competitions, and providing training and equipment for after-school sports programmes. Meanwhile, companies such as BT, Total and RBS (Royal Bank of Scotland) offer awards for schools, in the latter case specifically for those nominated by their employees; and, of course, technology companies like Microsoft, Apple and Promethean frequently provide 'free' equipment and software to schools. There are also companies such as Jazzy Books and Boomerang that produce school exercise and record books that incorporate advertising. Companies such as EdComms and Ten Nine, along with the organization Business in the Community, also serve as 'brokers' for such activities.

These more 'visible' dimensions of commercial influence are often controversial, and have been the focus of campaigns led by non-governmental organizations and teachers' unions.[2] Much of the criticism here has been fairly narrowly focused on the obesity issue, however: while the objection is ultimately to the principle of using schools as marketing venues, 'junk food' is currently a convenient high-profile target. Meanwhile, the UK government (the former Department of Children, Schools and Families) has produced guidelines on commercial 'partnerships', in collaboration with ISBA, the Incorporated Society of British Advertisers. These guidelines are broadly supportive of such activities, and place the burden on schools to assess whether they fulfil criteria to do with educational value and relevance – although in practice this may be far from straightforward to ascertain. School staff are urged to make judgements about the appropriateness of branding and sales messages, and to consider (for example in the case of voucher schemes) whether the terms of sale are sufficiently explicit. There are also specific guidelines relating to the promotion of HFSS foods, including regulations regarding vending machines in schools. Questions remain here, however, about how far schools are able to be proactive, confident partners in such relationships, or whether they are merely willing and compliant recipients of commercial *largesse* (Roberts, 1994).

A good instance of the sensitivity that surrounds more overt forms of marketing in UK schools in recent years was the Cadbury's 'Get Active!'

campaign, in which children were encouraged to collect tokens from chocolate bars which could then be exchanged for school sports equipment.[3] Campaigners estimated that children would need to consume £2000 worth of chocolate (around 1.25 million calories) in order to purchase just one of the items on offer, a set of volleyball posts.[4] Despite official government support, the scheme was quickly abandoned, although companies such as Nestlé and Kellogg's continue to sponsor sporting competitions and awards for schools (such as the Kellogg's Frosties Amateur Swimming Association Awards and its Football in the Community scheme, which provides coaching in schools: Wilkinson, 2006).

While the contradictions of the Cadbury's promotion were fairly obvious, other such schemes have been more successful. Walkers potato crisps (a division of Pepsi) ran its 'Books for Schools' campaign from 1999 to 2003, in association with Rupert Murdoch's News International, and apparently 'donated' £7 million worth of books to schools in exchange for tokens. The scheme was also endorsed by the government, and was described by Education Secretary David Blunkett as 'an excellent example of how business can get involved [in education] on a national level'.[5] A small-scale research study on the scheme (Waller, 1999) found that schools were not satisfied that the time and effort involved in gathering, cutting and sorting the tokens was well spent; and the choice of books was relatively narrow, being confined to one publishing house. There was also criticism of the fact that there was no co-operation between the company and teachers or school librarians – although there is no doubt that it increased the numbers of books in schools.

Given the political sensitivity surrounding child obesity, it is doubtful whether the Walkers scheme would have been sustained, although Nestlé (a familiar target for food campaigners) continues to run a similar 'Box Tops for Books' scheme, which also offers downloadable teaching resources.[6] A less controversial example would be Tesco's 'Computers for Schools' scheme, which has been running since 1992. It has undoubtedly played a key role in Tesco's attempts to offset criticism of its business practices and brand itself as a public-spirited company. The scheme has reportedly provided over £84 million worth of computers and computer-related goods to schools,[7] although the Consumers' Association (Which) has suggested that shoppers would need to spend around £220,000 in the store in order to collect enough vouchers for a £1,000 computer.[8]

Tesco's choice of computers as a focus for its activities in this area is, of course, symptomatic of the broader symbolic significance of technology in contemporary education. For decades, the marketing of computers has emphasized their status as an indispensable guarantee of educational relevance and credibility. As I have argued elsewhere (Buckingham, 2007), the involvement of technology companies in education has massively expanded on the back of assumptions about the 'information society' and the 'knowledge economy', and more recently in light of equally ill-defined notions of 'personalization' – despite the lack of good evidence from research that the use of such technology is effective, or even that it offers value for money compared with other approaches. In this state of digital euphoria, it has often been difficult to tell the difference between political (or indeed academic) advocates of 'technology-enhanced learning' and computer sales representatives. Computers in education are big business in themselves, as well as providing a powerful springboard into the domestic market, and the provision of sponsorship or 'free' equipment in schools is a powerful means for companies to build brand loyalty. With the advent of privately run digital 'learning platforms', which provide mutual surveillance between schools and homes, the marketing effectively becomes inescapable.

While such activities are certainly on the increase, there has been little independent critical evaluation of commercially sponsored educational resources themselves, or of the extent to which they are actually taken up in UK schools. Gary Raine (2007) presents the results of a survey of commercial activities specifically relating to health promotion in North of England primary schools. Over 50 per cent of the schools that responded had been involved in at least four types of commercial activity – voucher/token collection schemes (the most prevalent, at 85 per cent overall), commercial competitions or contests, business-linked sports coaching and sponsorship. Significantly, many of these activities were more commonly found in schools in more economically deprived areas (as is also the case in the US), suggesting that they function partly as a way of compensating for shortfalls in public provision. Very few of the schools had any clear policies on the issue, which would suggest that decisions are often made on an ad hoc basis. By comparison with studies undertaken in the late 1990s, Raine argues that these activities have grown in recent years, partly as a consequence of devolved budgets (so-called 'local management' of schools): while this has freed schools to operate independently in the market, it has also deprived them of the collective bargaining power that was formerly available through local authorities.

Such studies certainly show that companies are keen to use schools as a means of reaching the children's (and parents') market, not least because they seem to provide a 'captive audience' of some of the more elusive and hard-to-reach consumers. Whether such strategies are profitable – in the sense of giving shareholders a return on their investment – is perhaps another matter. The appearance of branded materials and equipment, and of forms of advertising, might be seen to imply endorsement of such products by schools; and while this approach might not necessarily prove effective with all students, it also addresses parents, who may be more inclined to accept it. However, there may also be a danger of schools appearing to give mixed messages, for example on issues such as nutrition and healthy eating, where corporate sponsorship may contradict the content of lessons (Raine, 2007); and, of course, there is the issue of bias, for example in the case of energy companies producing sponsored teaching materials about the environment (Schor, 2004), or banks and insurance companies providing curricula on 'financial literacy'.

It may be the case, as Wilkinson (2006) argues, that such activities contribute to the development of 'capitalistic world views and materialistic consumption' among students. However, it would be melodramatic to see this as a form of indoctrination into consumerism. Rather, the effects are likely to be more subtle and insidious. Kenway and Bullen's (2001) research in Australian schools suggests that students may be less attracted by in-school marketing than by the commercial appeals they encounter outside school, and in some cases may argue quite strongly against it, not least on ethical grounds. However, they may also come to see it as an inescapable fact of life, or a necessary means of getting 'something for free'. In this respect, the presence of commercial messages and brands may have become so ubiquitous as to be simply taken for granted, and any meaningful boundaries between the public and the private may have effectively ceased to exist.

Privatization: the rise of the education services industry

If the activities described thus far have, for the most part, been relatively visible, there are other forms of commercial involvement in education that have been much less apparent, at least to parents and children themselves. Stephen Ball (2007) has provided a detailed analysis of the growth of the UK 'education services industry', a sector that has expanded at a phenomenal pace in the past ten years. These companies are active in a very wide range of areas, at local, national and international levels: some are run for profit, although others are not. Their operations include: the 'contracted out' provision of educational goods and services, ranging from information technology to cleaning and school meals; the management and maintenance of school buildings and facilities; the sponsorship, governance and management of schools, groups of schools and entire education authorities; the provision of professional development and 'school improvement' services; the operation of inspection and advisory services; national programmes and strategies, such as the National Literacy and Numeracy strategies; examinations and assessment, and associated training and curriculum materials; and consultancy on local and national policy. There is often a powerful commercial synergy between these activities: in the UK, for example, privately owned examination boards have exclusive arrangements with commercial publishers on approved textbooks, as well as dominating the market in professional development courses. Numerous key government initiatives over the past ten years – such as Education Action Zones, Specialist Schools, Building Schools for the Future, the Private Finance Initiative and Academies – have included significant elements of commercial involvement. Key companies specializing in this sector include Serco, Jarvis, CEA, Nord Anglia and Capita, as well as major finance capital corporations such as HSBC and Goldman Sachs. Many of the companies involved here also have interests in other aspects of public service provision, including childcare and health services. As Ball (2004) indicates, some more entrepreneurial schools have also become independent players in this new market, selling their advice and services for profit to other schools.

Despite the extent of this form of commercial involvement, it has only tended to register on the public radar when there have been significant failures. In 2008, the chaotic mismanagement of the national SATs tests for 14-year-olds resulted in the government cancelling the contract it held with the US company ETS.[9] Other controversies have arisen around the government's Private Finance Initiative, in which school buildings are sold to private companies and then leased back; and in response to its flagship Academies programme, where private companies have paid relatively small amounts of money in exchange for taking control of the management and curriculum of schools, often in deprived inner-city areas (Fitz and Hafid, 2007). In general, however, the incremental and largely invisible nature of these developments has meant that they have effectively become 'naturalised' (Ball, 2008).

Ball sees these developments as symptomatic of much broader changes in the relationship between the state and the market that characterized New Labour's 'Third Way' and its efforts to compete in the globalized 'knowledge economy'. In education as in many other areas, the state is moving from being a provider of public services to being a commissioner or contractor, or a 'partner' with the private sector, while the private sector is widely believed to have superior expertise in terms of innovation, management and efficiency. In practice, however, many of the key personnel in the new education services industry are drawn from the (old) public sector, and the boundaries between the public and the private are extremely porous. Ball and Youdell's report for Education International (2008) also makes it clear that this is a global phenomenon, both in the sense that it involves global (or multinational) companies (such as Edison, ETS and GEMS), and also in that it is happening in many countries around the world. In such a context, insisting on a clear distinction or boundary line between the public and the private would seem to be an impossible – perhaps even utopian – task.

Marketization: schools as businesses

Beyond these various forms of commercialization and privatization, it is possible to identify another aspect of commercial influence in education, which might more aptly be termed *marketization*. This involves the importing of techniques and ideas from the private sector in order to make education more 'business-like'. It would include, for example, an emphasis on competition between schools and on parental choice, and a more corporate approach to the management of teaching staff. While these latter developments began in the UK under the Conservative governments of the 1980s, they gathered pace significantly under New Labour.

Advocates of marketization (e.g. Chubb and Moe, 1990; Tooley, 1994) make great play of the inflexibility and inefficiency of state provision, and assert that schooling can be more effectively organized according to the principles of the 'free market'. From this perspective, parents need to be able to function as rational economic agents, registering their choices in a competitive marketplace; and schools will simply adjust their offerings to meet demand. Marketization depends upon the existence of apparently objective metrics against which performance outputs can be calculated and compared. Thus, the quality of schools and of individual teachers is increasingly assessed in relation to pre-defined targets or standards; competition between schools proceeds on the basis of published league tables of test results, or 'report cards'; while parents are deemed to be able to use this information in choosing between schools for their children. Such developments implicitly define schools as though they were companies competing against each other in a free market, while parents are defined as customers or consumers of the services they provide (with children's learning, perhaps, as the product). In line with free-market ideology, this system follows the logic of the survival of the fittest: 'failing' schools, like failing companies, will either be publicly shamed into improving themselves, or simply cease to exist.

However, critics suggest that this belief in the effectiveness of a market model is largely based on faith (or ideology) rather than good evidence. They point out that there are many reasons why education cannot be organized as a 'pure' or perfectly competitive market system, even if one wished to do so (Ball, 1993; Lauder and Hughes, 1999): the matching of supply and demand is much more complex in the case of education than in the case of commodities, and schools cannot simply respond to demand in the nimble and flexible way that commercial businesses are imagined to do. In practice, the state is bound to intervene in order to regulate the market and to compensate for market failure.

Marketization is not a singular process, and its consequences for schools have been uneven and in some respects quite contradictory (Chitty, 1997). Over the past twenty years, new 'agents' (including managers, consultants and entrepreneurs of various kinds) have emerged in the education marketplace, and the working conditions and everyday practices of many teachers have altered dramatically. New categories of teaching and non-teaching staff have been created (advanced skills teachers, excellent teachers, teaching assistants) and new types of schools (grant maintained schools, Academies, specialist schools) have emerged. These shifts have been justified through new discourses, for example about modernization, efficiency and partnership. The changing role of parents is particularly notable here. In the first wave of marketization, parents were effectively redefined as 'customers', carefully scrutinizing the league tables, rather than as partners in their children's education (Bridges, 1994). In more recent years, as Hartley (2008) suggests, there has been a shift from a 'mass production' model to a more 'personalized' form of marketization, which is in line with the newer, more participatory approaches to marketing discussed in chapter 5. From this perspective, parents are no longer seen as 'mere consumers' but as active 'co-producers' of the services that are provided.

In the process, much more has come to depend upon how schools and teachers present and promote themselves. Schools are increasingly required to 'pitch' competitively for public funding, while teachers are assessed using approaches to performance management derived from the world of business. Head teachers are trained in entrepreneurial techniques, while some schools hire professional fundraisers to seek out corporate sponsorship. As Kenway and Bullen (2001) describe, schools are spending increasing amounts on corporate-style publicity, in the form of lavishly illustrated brochures, newsletters, websites and public relations materials directed at local media. Much greater attention is now paid to 'image work': the public areas of schools are frequently equipped in quasi-corporate style, there is considerable stress on 'smart' dress codes and personal appearance, and 'open days' for prospective parents are intensively stage-managed. Here again, the display of technology – computer suites, interactive whiteboards and other magical gadgets – is often crucial, although, as Kenway and Bullen suggest, appeals to forms of 'educational fundamentalism' – traditional values of discipline, academic achievement and career success – may also prove particularly powerful in the current climate. Yet while all schools are obligated to compete in this educational beauty contest, some are bound to remain significantly more attractive to consumers than others.

Implications for children

What have been the implications of these developments for children themselves? As in the parallel area of public broadcasting, the answer here is by no means straightforward. Hard evidence about whether these developments do in fact deliver what they promise is in short supply; and the question of what is to be measured (and how) is open to considerable dispute. As Stephen Ball (2007) suggests, it is important to avoid a simplistic polarization here between the public and the private – not least because this distinction has itself become so blurred through the developments I have described. Ball argues that there is no going back to a past in which 'monopoly public education' somehow worked efficiently and equitably in the interests of all: such a past never existed. However, like Cuban (2004), he also implies that such developments have had damaging consequences in terms of social equity, and have led to a narrowing of what is seen to count in terms of students' learning.

Ultimately, commercial companies' involvement in education is driven and made possible by the profit motive. While this may sometimes coincide with providing benefit to the 'customer', it does not necessarily always do so. Government schemes such as the Private Finance Initiative, for example, involve handing to private companies control of buildings and facilities that were previously in public ownership, and they can then be hired out for profit by such companies outside regular school hours. On the other hand, this has resulted in the improvement of existing schools and the building of new facilities that would almost certainly never have occurred otherwise.

Likewise, commercial involvement in school management has arguably resulted in greater funds being available to schools, albeit at some cost to their public mission. For example, sponsors of Academies do provide some funding, although in return they enjoy a considerable degree of control (for example, of key appointments, school governance, and to some extent the curriculum). Yet while there may be some kind of 'trade-off' here, it is hard to dispute the claim that these forms of privatization result in a significant reduction in local democratic accountability.

The marketization of education has had similarly ambivalent consequences. The government would certainly argue that the imposition of measurable targets and standards has served to drive up achievement overall; that parents are now significantly more 'empowered' in their relationships with schools; and that competition between schools has led to innovation and increased efficiency. However, for many families, perhaps particularly in cities, 'choice' depends principally on where one can afford to live, and, as such, it is largely a chimera in the first place. Studies point to the ways in which middle-class parents learn to 'play' local education markets to their own advantage (Ball, 2003). Oversubscribed schools are able to select the most 'teachable' students, who are predominantly middle-class, while working-class students are more frequently confined to schools that are deemed to be 'failing', and that struggle to avoid a spiral of decline (Lauder and Hughes, 1999). In this way, education markets systematically favour those who are already privileged in terms of social, educational and economic capital, and marketization would appear to result in an increasing degree of social segregation. Meanwhile, schools and teachers are bound to 'teach to the test' – sometimes almost cynically seeking to manipulate the statistics in order to secure competitive advantage in the league tables. None of this should be taken to imply a malevolent desire to increase inequality – on the contrary, it could well be seen as simply the inexorable logic of a market system.

Of course, there are complex processes at stake here, and it is important to separate the consequences of commercialization from those of privatization and of marketization – although this is not necessarily easy to do. Yet if we assess the consequences of these developments against the aims they were apparently designed to achieve, the story is by no means positive. Ball and Youdell (2008: 10) conclude that 'there is no clear-cut research based evidence demonstrating the benefits of programmes of school choice or contracting out of schools in terms of raising children's achievement'. A similar conclusion was reached by a House of Commons Select Committee in 2006 (Wilkinson, 2006: 257). Cuban's assessment of the situation in the United States is similarly sceptical, particularly in respect of evidence about long-term change (2004: 175); while Lauder and Hughes (1999) conclude, on the basis of extensive longitudinal research in New Zealand, that markets in education increase social polarization without delivering greater effectiveness or raising overall standards of achievement.

Of course, such conclusions can certainly be disputed: the evidence on such issues will probably never be definitive. Yet in some respects, the issue is rather broader than this. As Ball (2004) suggests, these processes may be part of a more general redefinition of what it means to be a teacher and a learner, which may in turn reflect broader shifts in the nature of human identity or subjectivity that some have seen as characteristic of 'late modern' societies (e.g. N. Rose, 1999). The 'logic' of the market appears to require both teachers and learners to behave in ever more individualistic, competitive ways, and yet also to engage in more intensive forms of self-regulation and self-surveillance. Ultimately, assessing the influence of commercial forces on education raises much broader political and philosophical questions about the kind of society we want: it is a matter of ethics and values, rather than something that can be assessed simply in terms of whether it improves efficiency or raises 'achievement'.

Learning outside school

The commercialization of educational goods and services has also been apparent outside schools. Again, this is by no means a new development. As Carmen Luke (1989) and others have pointed out, the modern 'invention' of childhood in the sixteenth and seventeenth centuries was accompanied by a whole range of pedagogic commodities aimed at parents and children, including primers, advice manuals and instructional books and playthings. Authors such as Ellen Seiter (1993), Stephen Kline (1993) and Gary Cross (1997) have shown that growth of the toy market in the early twentieth century was partly founded on beliefs about the developmental and educational value of play; and a sub-sector of the publishing and media industries has always subsisted on appealing to parents' educational aspirations for their children.

However, in recent years there has been a significant expansion in the market for broadly 'educational' toys, software, books and magazines targeted at the domestic consumer. There has been a proliferation of educational magazines, particularly aimed at pre-school children and their parents; the market for popular information books has become crowded with increasingly glossy and attractive new products; the sets of encyclopaedias countless children were bought in previous decades have now been largely superseded by CD-ROM versions; and, building on the faltering home software business, we are now seeing the emergence of a significant new market in online learning for domestic consumers (Buckingham and Scanlon, 2003, 2005). Perhaps the most remarkable manifestation of this phenomenon has been the boom in materials aimed at very young children – the *Baby Einstein* phenomenon, discussed in chapter 5.

In addition to educational materials, one can point to the growth of home tutoring (which is an entirely unregulated commercial market: see Ireson, 2004), and of lucrative franchises for supplementary out-of-school classes run by private companies such as Kumon, Crescendo and Stagecoach, both in mainstream curriculum subjects and in areas such as performing arts and sports. These phenomena are often linked to school provision: for example, many schools market revision guides (including those produced by commercially owned examination boards) or provide additional weekend or holiday programmes for 'gifted and talented' students run by commercial companies. As Allison Pugh (2009) suggests, wealthier parents are more able to control the environments in which their children grow up and the 'pathways' they follow (see chapter 8): they are able to address concerns about the perceived 'failure' of public schooling, and fears about the other children with whom their own might associate, either by buying private alternatives or by supplementing state provision with out-of-school 'enrichment' activities.

In seeking to capture this market, companies typically attempt to appeal to parents' 'better nature' – their sense of what they *should* be doing in order to qualify as Good Parents. This is perhaps most transparently the case with the marketing of home computers, which frequently involves claims about how they can 'help your child to get ahead' in the educational race (Nixon, 1998). Information technology, it is typically argued, will give children an 'educational edge' on the competition and help them 'move to the front of the class'. Likewise, the marketing of educational software to parents emphasizes its ability to 'make homework fun', and thereby enable the child to achieve better results at school (Buckingham et al., 2001). Such packages frequently contain 'assessment technology' that will enable parents to measure their child's progress in acquiring 'essential skills' and 'mastering fundamentals' – although this often sits awkwardly alongside claims about the 'magic' and 'enchantment' such software affords.

As Ball (2004) suggests, this kind of marketing typically speaks to parents' anxieties about competition – anxieties that are of course fuelled by contemporary developments in the marketization of schooling. In the individualistic 'risk society', prudent and responsible parents can no longer rely on state provision or on their own commonsense: they must look to the commercial market both for professional advice (for example in the growing range of specialized parenting magazines and websites) and in order to ensure that their child enjoys the opportunities and experiences that are increasingly seen to be essential for their future success. In this respect, this market can be seen as a further manifestation of what Lareau (2003) calls 'concerted cultivation' – a parenting style that positions the child as a kind of developmental project (see chapter 8). As Lareau and others suggest, this approach is most strongly manifested in the professional middle classes, who generally have the necessary financial resources to achieve it.

In practice, however, our research (e.g. Buckingham and Scanlon, 2003) suggests that there is often an awkward negotiation here, where children's wishes for play and entertainment tend to conflict with parents' interest in education – for example in struggles over how the home computer is used (see also Facer et al., 2003). Marketers try to square this circle with an emphasis on learning through play, or 'fun learning' – although the evidence suggests that this 'edutainment' strategy is one that tends to convince parents rather more easily than it does children. Certainly, there is good evidence that the educational promise of computers in the home is very far from being realized (Giacquinta et al., 1993; Kerawalla and Crook, 2005), and very little indication that these apparently 'educational' products are especially effective in terms of promoting learning.

Even so, these developments seem very likely to contribute to educational inequality. While such products and marketing appeals do attract parents from a range of social classes (see Buckingham and Scanlon, 2003), the fact remains that these opportunities are bound to be more available to children from affluent families. Indeed, the very existence of this market is likely to contribute to an atmosphere of growing educational competitiveness – and this is a competition in which poorer children will inevitably be further disadvantaged.

Leisure and play

The commercialization of children's out-of-school learning is paralleled by developments in their leisure and play. Sport, play and leisure spaces are increasingly becoming sites for commercial promotion, and facilities that were formerly publicly owned and run are steadily being privatized (see

France et al., 2009). As we have seen (chapter 8), children's leisure has become steadily more 'domesticated' or home-based. At least in the UK, children are now much more confined to their homes, and much less independently mobile, than they were thirty years ago (Valentine, 2004). Since the 1970s, 'playing out' in the street or in open spaces has steadily been displaced by domestic entertainment (particularly via television and computers) and – especially among more affluent classes – by supervised leisure activities such as organized sports, music lessons and so forth. Meanwhile, the availability of public play areas has reduced, both in towns – where population density has increased – and in the countryside – where agri-business has rendered large areas less accessible. Formerly public leisure services are being contracted out, and private companies are also increasingly the ones providing key services. If children have to 'pay to play' outside the home, new social inequalities are bound to emerge.

One contemporary development that is especially relevant to younger children is the expansion of commercialized play spaces that provide soft play areas, 'ball parks', climbing frames and safe surfaces. Corporate providers such as Tumbletots, Charlie Chalks and Wacky Warehouses have been quick to recognize the emerging opportunities to engage children in more challenging forms of play, but in a safe environment. Such commercial play spaces also seek to accentuate their attractiveness to parents, since it is ultimately parents who are the main 'consumers': they may be linked to shops or pubs, or provide coffee mornings where parents can meet each other while their children play. Indeed, it has been argued that children occupy only a marginal role in the production of these play environments, and in contributing to the decision to use them; and, as such, these spaces provide more for the needs of adults than those of children (McKendrick et al., 2000).

Theme parks, the contemporary successors to amusement parks, are also now a major leisure destination for families with children. Since 1955 when Disneyland opened its first theme park, with entertainment and fairground rides built entirely around the company's products, corporations have increasingly been creating dedicated branded spaces that combine pleasure with promotion. Other brands have secured spaces within larger theme park complexes by sponsoring popular rides and locations, and companies have also played an increasing role in sponsoring and branding exhibits in settings such as museums, zoos and 'heritage industry' attractions. The combination of entertainment and consumption is also characteristic of major shopping malls. Centres such as Bluewater, the largest complex in the South-east of England, typically claim to be 'much more than just a shopping destination'. Bluewater contains a multiplex cinema, numerous restaurants and eating places, together with play areas specifically designed for children, including a climbing wall. This integration of shopping and play is also apparent in stores stocking children's products. The Lego brand stores and the more 'educationally' branded Early Learning Centre, for example, provide extensive opportunities for play with their products, while this same logic is applied in other public spaces, as with Electronic Arts' provision of video games for bored children waiting with parents in airport lounges (France et al., 2009).

Here again, the commercial market may well be providing greater opportunities for leisure and play, but most of them are much more readily available to children from more wealthy families. As a result, it may be that disadvantaged children are more likely to be confined to the home, which could in turn have implications for their physical health, not least in respect of obesity. Alternatively, disadvantaged children might be more likely to resort to playing or socialising with each other in public spaces – or in commercial spaces such as shopping malls – where they may be more readily perceived as 'causing trouble', and hence come under increasing surveillance.

Consumer education and media literacy

I have argued in this chapter that schools – and education more broadly – have become increasingly inextricable from the operations of the commercial market. It might seem paradoxical, then, to suggest that they can also provide opportunities for developing a more critical view of consumer culture. One might well argue that commercial imperatives and corporate values have so thoroughly colonized public education that no escape seems possible: only a radical recovery of the public mission of the school would suffice. My own view is rather more sanguine, or perhaps pragmatic. I would argue that schools (and indeed parents) can play a crucial role in enabling children to understand and to critique the operations of the commercial market, and if necessary to resist them.

There is a long history of attempts at 'consumer education', not all of which have been very successful. Lisa Jacobson (2004) describes initiatives in US schools in the 1920s and 1930s, undertaken partly with the collaboration of banks, which were designed to promote frugal spending and good saving habits. These forms of 'thrift education' gradually gave way to less restrictive and moralistic programmes of 'consumer training', although there is little evidence that either approach was especially effective.

Today, 'consumer education' is often understood in similarly functional terms, as a matter of becoming a 'wise consumer'. Ofcom, the UK media regulator, for example, has defined 'consumer literacy' as 'the ability to choose and use communications products effectively' (Bowe, 2007) – suggesting a view of the consumer as an essentially rational economic agent.

Alternatively, consumer education can be seen as a matter of informing consumers about their rights – for instance in relation to deceptive or intrusive practices – and about how to prevent or complain about them. For example, in England, consumer education is a dimension of the National Curriculum for Citizenship, where it focuses primarily on consumers' 'rights and responsibilities'. The government's Office of Fair Trading sees consumer education as a means of creating 'empowered' consumers, who will demand high standards from business and thereby promote vigorous and competitive markets (Office of Fair Trading, 2004). More narrowly, there have been initiatives designed to promote 'financial literacy', or 'financial capability', which refers largely to the ability to retrieve, understand and evaluate information about financial products and services: such initiatives have been promoted in the UK by the financial services regulator, the Financial Services Authority, and internationally by the Organisation for Economic Co-operation and Development. Personal finance education is also part of the English National Curriculum for Personal, Social and Health Education (PSHE).

While such initiatives are broadly positive, they are often quite narrowly defined. In general, they seek to encourage young people to become well-informed, rational and prudent consumers – an approach which would seem to neglect the non-rational, expressive and symbolic aspects of consumption that theorists have seen as increasingly significant in the contemporary world (see chapter 2). The inconsistent positioning of consumer education within the curriculum also reflects an awkward tension between consumption and citizenship: it betrays an uncertainty about whether consumption is simply a matter for the individual, or a broader question of social practices and values (Benn, 2004).

By contrast, Kenway and Bullen (2001) propose a much more ambitious approach to what they call 'consumer-media education'. Their broader argument here is that, for many students, school now lacks the 'enchantment' offered by consumer culture, and that as a result it is typically confined to 'the periphery of their identities and concerns'. Schools need to engage critically with consumer culture, but in doing so they need to beware of appearing moralistic and authoritarian, and of the limitations of rationalistic critique. On the contrary, they need to address the emotional, aesthetic and embodied dimensions of young people's engagement with consumer culture: 'consumer-media education' needs to incorporate elements of play and pleasure, as well as politics. For Kenway and Bullen, understanding consumer culture therefore involves much more than prudent budgeting and clever shopping: it also entails a profound reflection on one's emotional investments in consumption, and its role in terms of identity and 'life politics'.

While these authors do provide a few suggestions as to how this might be achieved in practice, their proposals for what they call 'a pedagogy of the profane and the popular' are somewhat nebulous. However, such issues have frequently been addressed in a more concrete way in the field of media literacy education. Although a detailed account of this approach is beyond the scope of this book (see Buckingham, 2003), it is important to emphasize that media education can go well beyond developing children's critical understanding of advertising. For example, most Media Studies courses include a component investigating the media industries, which will often include student-led research and simulations of industry practice. This kind of work can provide important opportunities for children to learn about, and to reflect on, the ways in which commercial forces determine the kinds of entertainment and information that are available to them. Media education also involves both critical study and creative production of media; and it is in the latter area that students can be enabled to explore and analyse the more emotional and symbolic aspects of their engagement with consumer culture.

Of course, this is not to say that media educators have solved all the problems that are potentially at stake here: media education can be just as rationalistic and instrumental – and sometimes as politically self-righteous – as more mainstream approaches (Buckingham, 1998). The advent of more 'participatory' marketing practices also poses further difficulties for media educators. Our research (Skaar et al., 2010) suggests that teachers themselves may be unaware of the nature and extent of digital marketing to children, and that existing classroom strategies (such as the textual 'deconstruction' of advertisements) may be less than effective in addressing this. More significantly, the ways in which contemporary marketing is implicated in children's peer-group relationships – for example in the area of social networking sites – may make it particularly challenging for teachers to deal with.

However, it is important to stress that media education is not primarily conceived as a form of protection or inoculation against media influence.

As we have seen (chapter 3), people (adults or children) who are more media literate are not necessarily less immune to media influence. Yet the primary aim of media literacy education is not to reduce the influence of 'bad' media or advertising, any more than the aim of literacy education is to reduce the influence of 'bad' books. Rather, it should be seen as part of a more fundamental rethinking of how we teach about culture and communication in a world that is increasingly saturated with commercial media. As such, education in this area should not be seen as an alternative to regulation of the market, but as a necessary accompaniment to it.

Conclusion

In broad terms, it is relatively easy to establish the growing scale and nature of commercial involvement in education. Yet it is significantly harder to identify its implications for children. One could argue that (as in other areas) the growing involvement of commercial companies has made available a range of new products, facilities and services that might not otherwise have been provided. Yet whether or not they meet the needs of children, parents and teachers, and whether or not they make a positive contribution to learning, depends on how these things are defined.

The issues addressed in this chapter and the previous one are potentially much more broad-ranging than those relating primarily to advertising and marketing. Commercial forces are playing an ever more important role in determining the kinds of opportunities and experiences that are now available to children and young people. Commercial companies are increasingly key players in the provision of public services. Even where the private sector is not directly involved, the commercial market has become the model for how such services will be organized and delivered. Children's access to learning, play and leisure experiences is now, more than ever, a market opportunity – and, as such, some children are bound to be more able to enjoy and benefit from these things than others. In the process, notions of the public good are effectively being replaced by the principle of customer satisfaction.

I have concentrated on two domains here – broadcasting and education – but this analysis could certainly be extended to other domains, such as the provision of health and social care. These developments may represent gains as well as losses for children. Ultimately, however, the market is almost bound to accentuate existing inequalities. It is to this issue, and its broader implications for public policy, that I turn in my concluding chapter.

12

Conclusion: living in a material world

The growing concern about children's consumption that I have addressed in this book is partly a response to changing circumstances. In recent years, children have become an increasingly important market in their own right. Companies are now targeting children more energetically than ever before, and at an ever-younger age; and they are using a range of new tactics, at least some of which raise important ethical concerns. Although there is a long history of commercial marketing to children, its current scope and intensity are quite unprecedented. Meanwhile, commercial forces have also become significantly more influential in the provision of public goods and services, including education and leisure opportunities. The privatization and marketization of schools have led to newly 'consumerized' approaches to teaching and learning; fundamental values of parental care and belonging have increasingly come to be expressed through the purchasing and use of commercial goods and services; and consumption has played an increasingly important role in how children construct their peer group relationships.

This issue is obviously important in its own right, but it has also come to serve as a focus for a whole range of other concerns, at least some of which are only marginally related to it. As we have seen, there is a tendency in popular debate to regard children as merely incompetent victims of exploitation. As is ever the case, the focus on children provides campaigners with a powerful means of commanding public assent. Childhood, they tell us, is being commercialized, children's innocence is being corrupted, and the modern world has degenerated into an empty, materialistic hell. Anyone who dares to question such claims clearly could not care less about children.

Part of my aim in this book has been to offer a corrective to such melodramatic views. I do not regard children as merely passive or incompetent consumers. I believe that claims about the power of advertising and marketing are often absurdly exaggerated. I have challenged moralistic arguments that seek to blame children (and indeed parents) for apparently surrendering to trivial, materialistic desires. I have questioned our familiar tendency as adults to stigmatize children's consumption – as excessive, as tasteless, as necessarily harmful – in ways that we assume our own consumption is not. To this extent, my approach might be seen as giving support to the rhetoric (if not necessarily the practice) of some children's marketers – although I have cast an equally sceptical eye on the superficial, and to some extent rather hypocritical, assertions of the brand gurus.

However, my broader aim has been to move beyond the polarized terms in which this issue is typically discussed. Children are not *either* passive victims *or* empowered and autonomous social actors. Consumption is not simply a matter of manipulation and control *or* of choice and freedom. Consumers are not simply 'slaves to the brand', but nor are they joyfully creating their own meanings – let alone expressing resistance to the powers that be. Such arguments on both sides appear to fall prey to a kind of easy sentimentality, whether that is expressed as grandiose intellectual pessimism or as a kind of postmodern wishful thinking.

In moving beyond this easy polarization, I have sought to reframe the whole issue of children's consumption. This is partly a matter of seeing consumption in context. Thus, I have attempted to locate the growth of the children's market within a broader social and historical context – not least of significant shifts in family life. I have argued that we must see children's consumption – and, by extension, adults' consumption as well – not in individualistic terms, but as embedded within relationships with parents and peers, and with the wider community. It is partly through their consumption practices that children build connections with the people around them, and participate in the social world: identity or subjectivity is inevitably produced within consumer culture. Ultimately, this makes it very difficult to distinguish between commercial and non-commercial activities, or between consumer practices and a 'social context' that is somehow *not* about consumption.

To this extent, then, the narrative of the 'commercialization of childhood' is at least an oversimplification. Children's growing access to consumer goods and services is part of the much broader historical development of consumer capitalism over the past several centuries. The market has not somehow invaded or colonized the sacred space of childhood: for better and worse, children are born into a world of commodities. In a capitalist economy, childhood (like adulthood) does not and cannot exist outside of market relations. And yet we persist in talking as though consumption were somehow separate from life, rather than something that is unavoidably embedded within our most mundane and most intimate social practices.

In addition to questioning the terms of the public debate, I have also challenged some of the academic research in this area. I have questioned psychological accounts, which tend to measure children's development as consumers simply in terms of their alignment with adult norms. I have especially challenged the methods and assumptions of 'effects' research, which I see as providing a fatally reductive account of the social world. By contrast, I have argued for a cultural studies approach, which takes account not only of the perspectives and activities of consumers but also of the operations of the market, and of the relations between them. Such an approach moves us beyond the theoretical dichotomy between structure and agency, and offers the potential for a more dynamic, contextual approach.

I have also argued that a narrow focus on advertising or marketing obscures the complexity of children's relations with the commercial world. Expenditure on advertising is now only a small part of total marketing budgets, and, as the most visible and obvious aspect of marketing, it is also the easiest for children to understand. In interpreting children's consumption, we need to look at the broader landscape, not only of marketing and promotion but also of the chain of production, distribution and supply. We also need to address the changing relations between the public and the private. Privatization and marketization have become the unquestioned shibboleths of contemporary neo-liberal societies. Few politicians now seem prepared to question the assumption that the market is more effective than the state in providing for people's needs. Indeed, at the time of writing (mid-2010), the UK has a new coalition government that seems intent on using economic difficulties as a kind of alibi for a wholesale dismantling of public services.

Yet, in broad terms, a market system is bound to result in increasing inequality. Of course, this is essentially to do with employment and the effect on family earnings, rather than with the market in goods and services per se. Even so, these inequalities then lead to large differences in how lucrative different households are for businesses. This has become even more apparent as we have moved from 'mass' to 'niche' markets, and as marketers have increasingly been able to analyse the value of different customers and target the most valuable. This is bound to mean that the needs of the less affluent are less well served, and this might in turn be expected to lead to significant consequences in terms of physical and mental health. For example, it has demonstrably led to phenomena such as 'food deserts', and the general decline of neighbourhood commerce in working-class communities (Chin, 2001).

As such, one might expect that children from less affluent backgrounds would experience lower levels of mental wellbeing (however this is defined). Yet this is not straightforwardly the case. For example, it is by no means clear that children living in poorer families experience greater mental health problems than those from more affluent backgrounds, or are more likely to come into conflict with their parents or peers – or indeed that they are more 'materialistic'. There is a danger in some of the debate on these issues of pathologizing the consumption of poorer families. The poor are regarded as bad consumers, deluded by marketing to want things they cannot have, and to want things that are worthless in any case. If they suffer in this situation, then it is essentially their own fault. Yet research suggests that poorer children may in fact be *less* 'materialistic', in the sense that they learn to adjust and limit their desires in light of what they know they are likely to get – and in relation to the needs of others (see Chin, 2001; Ridge, 2002).

Some have argued that the crucial issue here is to do with the gap between aspiration and reality: if you are constantly reminded that other people have more than you, then you are more likely to be unhappy (Layard, 2005). Certainly, there is little doubt that parents in less wealthy families experience greater difficulty in dealing with their children's demands for consumer goods. Parents may be more inclined to go without things themselves in order to provide for their children; and children and parents may feel there is greater pressure to buy expensive goods (such as 'designer' clothing) in order to disguise the stigma of poverty – although, in this sense, consumption might be seen as a focus for *resistance* to inequality, and to the indignity and injury it imposes. Among upwardly mobile families, and in a general context of rising affluence, there may also be a generational effect. Such parents may have difficulty coming to terms with the fact that their children have greater access to material goods than they did themselves in their own childhood: they may want to give them 'the things we never had', but they may also experience considerable ambivalence and guilt about this.

This would suggest that the issue is more to do with relative deprivation than absolute deprivation – that is, with inequality rather than with poverty per se. As we have seen, the significance of material goods (or the lack of them) depends heavily upon social comparison – both with others who are more or less wealthy than oneself, and with one's previous experience, and that of other family members. Being poor feels worse if you know that other people are better-off; and you may be likely to want things more if you know you cannot have them. By offering people images of what they cannot have, and stimulating the desire for such things, consumer culture could thus be seen to exacerbate the existing pressures of living in poverty.

Framing the issue in this way offers some alternatives in terms of policy and social action. This is not the place to explore the detail of possible policy initiatives – not least because these are so contingent upon immediate circumstances.[1] Yet here again, there is a need to take a broader view. Banning advertising to children – which seems to be an obsessive preoccupation among some campaigners – is unlikely to make a significant difference to anything (except perhaps the profits of advertising agencies), and would also raise a whole host of legal and logistical problems. Of course, there is a continuing need for regulation – and particularly, at the moment, for some tighter regulation of digital marketing (to adults as well as children). It also makes good sense to use education as a means of developing children's critical understanding of the operations of the commercial market – although not if education is regarded merely as a form of inoculation, or a source of moralistic warnings about evil marketers.

However, we also need to consider what is at stake in talking about children in the first place. Adults are susceptible to many of the same processes of commercial influence and persuasion as children. As I have shown, parents are profoundly implicated in children's consumption, since consumption has come to carry meanings of love and care, and of longing and nostalgia. Like children, adults routinely use commodities as means of claiming power and status, of finding emotional security and identity, and even of expressing resistance to authority. And yet we persist in talking as though children were the problem – as though children were somehow uniquely 'at risk', and as though regulating their access to knowledge and power in respect of the market would somehow solve this problem. Yet as Ellen Seiter (1993) has argued, the idea that children can be somehow sheltered from consumption is a peculiarly middle-class delusion – one which fuels its own specialized consumer markets in 'quality' toys and 'educational' services.

Ultimately, we need to avoid confusing symptoms and causes here. The key problem with the contemporary 'moral panics' about children's consumption – for instance in relation to obesity and 'sexualization' – is that they distract attention from the complexity and difficulty of real social problems. As with the debates about media violence, multidimensional social issues become reduced to a simple cause-and-effect logic; and blaming the media becomes an easy way for politicians to look as though they are 'doing something' in response to public concern. In the process, deeper underlying causes are typically neglected. Blaming the bad effects of capitalism on marketing to children may be therapeutic for some, but it is ultimately superficial and misguided.

As I have argued, it is the historical coming together of several forms of social change – the extension of capitalist markets, but also changes in family life, moves towards privatization, and rising inequality – that have combined to make the issue of children's relation with the commercial market significantly more acute. These changes have not been consistent in their effects, nor are they inexorable. Yet it is these issues that we need to understand and address if we really want to do something about children's consumption.

Notes

1 Exploited or empowered? Constructing the child consumer

1 News stories relating to these events may be found at: http://news.bbc.co.uk/1/hi/
scotland/2579137.stm and www.telegraph.co.uk/news/uknews/5732821/Parents
-banned-from-sports-day-over-paedophile-fears.html.

2 See www.independent.co.uk/news/education/education-news/authors-boycott
-schools-over-sexoffence-register-1748267.html.

3 See www.telegraph.co.uk/news/yourview/1528718/Daily-Telegraph-campaign-to-halt
-death-of-childhood.html.

4 See, for example, www.timesonline.co.uk/printFriendly/0,,1-2-363060,00.html (23 July
2002); and www.archbishopofcanterbury.org/651 (interview on the BBC *Today*
programme, 13 December 2006).

2 Understanding consumption

1 I participated in this myself at the time: see Buckingham (1993a); and, in response to
Willis, Buckingham (1993b).

2 *Grumpy Old Men* is an ironic TV show in the UK featuring men of a certain age
complaining endlessly about their pet hates of modern life. There is a *Grumpy Old
Women* as well.

5 The contemporary children's market

1 Liverpool Victoria Friendly Society (2010). Childcare and education account for over
half of this amount, although private school fees are not included.

2 These figures come from submissions to the Children's Society Good Childhood
Enquiry, Lifestyle Theme (2007); and the Office of National Statistics.

6 The fear of fat: obesity, food and consumption

1 Kim Severson, 'Obesity "a threat" to US security: Surgeon General urges cultural shift',
San Francisco Chronicle 7 January 2003: www.sfgate.com/cgi-bin/article
.cgi?f=/c/a/2003/01/07/MN166871.DTL.

2 It is notable that the more alarming projections of the UK government's Foresight
report (2007) have recently been revised downwards. See 'Child obesity forecasts
"excessive" says report', *Guardian* 3 November 2009: www.guardian.co.uk/
society/2009/nov/03/child-obesity-levelling-off.

3 This in itself points to an unexplained flaw in the argument: if HFSS advertising was
declining prior to the new regulations, and yet obesity was rising, this would suggest
that the relationship between them is far from straightforward.

4   It should be emphasized that, while overall diets might be considered 'healthy' or 'unhealthy', this distinction cannot meaningfully be applied to specific foods in themselves, even if it routinely is.

5   As Martyn Richmond (pers.comm., Ph.D. research in progress, Institute of Education, University of London, 2010) has pointed out, the element of playful 'rebellion' here continues in later childhood and young adulthood, not least in the phenomenon of 'binge drinking' and substance use, and more generally in the habitual consumption of 'unhealthy' treats.

6   M. Richmond, pers. comm.

7   Too much, too soon? Marketing, media and the sexualization of girls

1   For examples, see www.dailymail.co.uk/news/article-412195/Tesco-condemned-selling -pole-dancing-toy.html; www.gazetteseries.co.uk/uk_national_news/4668497.Tight_ trousers__too_sexy__at_school/; http://women.timesonline.co.uk/tol/life_and_style/ women/families/article6910040.ece.

2   See, for example, http://news.bbc.co.uk/1/hi/8521403.stm; http://www.mumsnet. com/campaigns/let-girls-be-girls; and on Cameron's comments, http://news.bbc.co. uk/1/hi/8521403.stm and www.dailymail.co.uk/debate/article-1252156/DAVID-CAMERON-Sexualisation-children-too-young.html.

3   The original design for Barbie was reportedly based on an image of a prostitute in a German adult cartoon (Clark, 2007: 111).

4   For instance, the age of consent in Japan is currently 13.

5   A fuller critique of these reports, and of the media effects literature in this area, may be found in Buckingham et al. (2010).

8   Rethinking 'pester power': children, parents and consumption

1   The following sections draw on two reviews undertaken by the Social Issues Research Centre for our assessment of 'The Impact of the Commercial World on Children's Wellbeing' (Social Issues Research Centre, 2009a, 2009b). These reviews draw in turn on a range of sources, including the Office of National Statistics, the General Household Survey, the UK Census, the Annual Population Survey, the British Social Attitudes Survey, the United Kingdom Time Use Survey, and others.

2   It should be noted that such codes do not currently apply to aspects of online marketing such as 'wish lists' on internet shopping sites, at least in the UK.

3   The use of structural equation modelling is especially confusing in this context. Buijzen and her colleagues use the technical term 'path' to define an association between variables; yet the term 'path' in everyday language might well be assumed to imply a direction of causality, which in this case it does not.

4   There is an unstated social class dimension to this distinction, which is apparent when one compares such psychological studies with sociological accounts of parenting, for example the work of Lareau (2003).

5   There are strong echoes here of Ellen Seiter's (1999) studies, which found that middle-class parents were much more dismissive towards popular television, and much more inclined to express concern about its allegedly harmful effects, than working-class parents. The same differences were apparent in the attitudes of teachers and care-workers serving the different groups.

9   Beyond 'peer pressure': consumption and identity in the peer group

1   There are some parallels here with Ellen Seiter's (2003) arguments about the ways in which children's media culture excludes adults, discussed in chapter 3.

2   See Mintel (2010) 'Supermarket sweeps up childrenswear sales' – www.mintel.com/press-centre/press-releases/488/supermarket-sweeps-up-childrenswear-sales.
3   Ibid.

10   Screening the market: the case of children's television

1   In addition to the sources cited, this section draws on work undertaken with my student Rachel Bailey: see Bailey (2010).

11   Consuming to learn – learning to consume: education goes to market

1   The campaigning website www.obligation.org provides copious information on such activities.
2   Examples in the UK would include the charity Baby Milk Action, which publishes a teaching pack *Seeing through the Spin*; and the National Union of Teachers, which publishes critical guidance on the use of commercial teaching materials. Meanwhile, there is a Campaign for Commercial-Free Education in Ireland, and an International Day of Action Against the Commercialization of Education is apparently being planned.
3   www.cadbury.co.uk/EN/CTB2003/talk_to_us/faq/getactive_debate.htm.
4   www.foodcomm.org.uk/cadbury_03.htm.
5   www.brandrepublic.com/news/478730/superbrands-case-studies-walkers/.
6   www.boxtops4education.co.uk/home.aspx.
7   www.computersforschools.co.uk/: this has since mutated into a programme involving sports equipment as well as computers.
8   http://news.bbc.co.uk/2/hi/uk_news/education/1694388.stm.
9   www.guardian.co.uk/education/2008/aug/15/sats.schools.

12   Conclusion: living in a material world

1   Our government report (Buckingham et al., 2009) provides a fairly substantial discussion of potential policy responses, in terms of both regulation and education. Undertaken in the dying days of Gordon Brown's ill-fated administration, its arguments here would certainly need to be rethought in light of the subsequent change of government – and, indeed, of the impact of global recession.

References

Acuff, D. S. and Reiher, R. H. (2005) *Kidnapped: How Irresponsible Marketers are Stealing the Minds of Your Children* Chicago: Dearborn

Aksglaede, L., Olsen, L. W., Sorensen, T. and Juul, A. (2008) 'Forty year trends in timing of pubertal growth spurt in 157,000 Danish school children', *PLoS One* 3(7): e2728

Alanen, L. (2001) 'Explorations in generational analysis', in L. Alanen and B. Mayall (eds.) *Conceptualizing Child–Adult Relations* London: Routledge Falmer

Aldridge, A. (2003) *Consumption* Cambridge: Polity

Ambler, T. (2006) 'Does the UK promotion of food and drink to children contribute to their obesity?' *International Journal of Advertising* 25(2): 137–56

American Psychological Association (2004) *Report of the APA Task Force on Advertising and Children* Washington, DC: APA

American Psychological Association (2007) *Report of the APA Task Force on the Sexualization of Girls* Washington, DC: APA

Arthurs, J. (2004) *Television and Sexuality* Buckingham: Open University Press

Arvidsson, A. (2006) *Brands: Meaning and Value in Media Culture* London: Routledge

Ashley, B., Hollows, J., Jones, S. and Taylor, B. (2004) *Food and Cultural Studies* London: Routledge

Attwood, F. (2007) 'Sexed up: theorizing the sexualization of culture', *Sexualities* 9(1): 77–94

Attwood, F. (2009) *Mainstreaming Sex: The Sexualisation of Western Culture* London: I. B.Tauris

Australian Senate (2007) *Inquiry into the Sexualisation of Children in the Contemporary Media Environment* www.aph.gov.au/Senate/committee/eca_ctte/sexualisation_of_children/tor.htm

Bailey, R. (2010) 'UK children's television brands in the 00s'. Associateship Report, Institute of Education, University of London

Ball, S. (1993) 'Education markets, choice and social class: the market as a class strategy in the UK and the US', *British Journal of Sociology of Education* 14(1): 3–19

Ball, S. (2003) *Class Strategies and the Education Market: The Middle Classes and Social Advantage* London: Routledge

Ball, S. (2004) 'Education for sale! The commodification of everything?' Annual Education Lecture, Department of Education and Professional Studies, King's College London

Ball, S. (2007) *Education Plc: Understanding Private Sector Participation in Public Sector Education* London: Routledge

Ball, S. (2008) 'The legacy of ERA, privatization and the policy ratchet', *Educational Management, Administration and Leadership,* 36(2): 185–99

Ball, S. and Youdell, D. (2008) *Hidden Privatisation in Public Education* Brussels: Education International

Banerjee, R. and Dittmar, H. (2008) 'Individual differences in children's materialism: the role of peer relations', *Personality and Social Psychology Bulletin* 34: 17–31

Banet-Weiser, S. (2004) ' "We pledge allegiance to kids": Nickelodeon and citizenship', in H. Hendershot (ed.) *Nickelodeon Nation: The History, Politics and Economics of America's Only TV Channel for Kids* New York: New York University Press

Banet-Weiser, S. (2007) *Kids Rule! Nickelodeon and Consumer Citizenship* Durham, NC: Duke University Press

Barber, B. (2007) *Consumed: How Markets Corrupt Children, Infantilize Adults, and Swallow Citizens Whole* New York: Norton

Barker, M. (1984) *A Haunt of Fears* London: Pluto

Barthes, R. (1990) *The Fashion System* Berkeley: University of California Press

Barwise, P., Young, B., Livingstone, S. and Buckingham, D. (2009) 'Children, commerce and obesity: what role does marketing play?' Technical Appendix to Buckingham *The Impact of the Commercial World on Children's Wellbeing* London: Department of Children, Schools and Families and Department of Culture, Media and Sport

Basham, P., Gori, G. and Luik, J. (2006) *Diet Nation: Exploring the Obesity Crusade* London: Social Affairs Unit

Bauman, Z. (2007) *Consuming Life* Cambridge: Polity

Beardsworth, A. and Keil, T. (1998) *Sociology on the Menu* London: Routledge

Benn, J. (2004) 'Consumer education between "consumership" and citizenship: experiences from studies of young people', *International Journal of Consumer Studies* 28(2): 108–16

Bennett, T., Savage, M., Silva, E. B., Warde, A., Gayo-Cal, M. and Wright, D. (2009) *Culture, Class, Distinction* London: Routledge

Best, J. (1990) *Threatened Children* Chicago: University of Chicago Press

Best, J. (ed.) (1994) *Troubling Children: Studies of Children and Social Problems* New York: Aldine de Gruyter

Blumler, J. (1992) *The Future of Children's Television in Britain* London: Broadcasting Standards Council

Blumler, J. and Biltereyst, D. (1998) *The Integrity and Erosion of Public Television for Children: A Pan-European Survey* London: Broadcasting Standards Commission

Bocock, R. (1993) *Consumption* London: Routledge

Boden, S. (2006a) 'Another day, another demand: how parents and children negotiate consumption matters', *Sociological Research Online* 11(2) www.socresonline.org.uk/11/2/boden.html

Boden, S. (2006b) 'Dedicated followers of fashion? The influence of popular culture on children's social identities', *Media, Culture and Society* 28(2): 289–98

Bolton, R. N. (1983) 'Modeling the impact of television food advertising on children's diets', *Current Issues and Research in Advertising* 6(1): 173–99

Born, G. (2004) *Uncertain Vision: Birt, Dyke and the Reinvention of the BBC* London: Secker and Warburg

Bourdieu, P. (1979) *Distinction: A Social Critique of the Judgment of Taste* London: Routledge and Kegan Paul

Bowe, C. (2007) *What is Consumer Literacy and Why Does It Matter?* London: Ofcom Consumer Panel

Bragg, S. and Buckingham, D. (2002) *Young People and Sexual Content on Television: A Review of the Research* London: Broadcasting Standards Commission

Bragg, S. and Buckingham, D. (forthcoming) 'Global concerns and local negotiations: mothers, daughters and the sexualisation of childhood debate', submitted to *Feminist Media Studies*

Brandtzaeg, P. (2009) 'Norwegian children's experiences of cyberbullying', *Journal of Children and Media* 3(4): 349–63

Bridges, D. (1994) 'Parents: customers or partners?' in D. Bridges and T. McLaughlin (eds.) *Education and the Market Place* London: Falmer

Bromley, H. (2004) 'Localizing Pokémon through narrative play', in J. Tobin (ed.) *Pikachu's Global Adventure: The Rise and Fall of Pokémon* Durham, NC: Duke University Press

Brooks, L. (2006) *The Story of Childhood: Growing Up in Modern Britain* London: Bloomsbury

Brougère, G. (2004) 'How much is a Pokémon worth: Pokémon in France', in J. Tobin (ed.) *Pikachu's Global Adventure: The Rise and Fall of Pokémon* Durham, NC: Duke University Press

Brown, H. (2006) *Parenting for Dummies* Chichester: John Wiley

Brown, J. D., White, A. B. and Nickopoulou, L. (1993) 'Disinterest, intrigue, resistance: early adolescent girls' use of sexual media content', in B. S. Greenberg, J. D. Brown and N. L. Buerkel-Rothfuss (eds.) *Media, Sex and the Adolescent* Cresskill, NJ: Hampton Press

Brusdal, R. (2008) 'Little emperors in an affluent society'. Keynote address, Child and Teen Consumption Conference, Trondheim, Norway, 24–25 April

Bryman, A. (1995) *Disney and his Worlds* London: Routledge

Bucholtz, M. (2007) 'Shop talk: branding, consumption and gender in American middle-class youth interaction', in B. S. McElhinny (ed.) *Words, Worlds, and Material Girls: Language, Gender, Globalization* Berlin: de Gruyter

Buckingham, D. (1993a) *Children Talking Television* London: Falmer

Buckingham, D. (1993b) 'Rereading audiences', in D. Buckingham (ed.) *Reading Audiences: Young People and the Media* Manchester: Manchester University Press

Buckingham, D. (1993c) 'Boys' talk: television and the policing of masculinity', in D. Buckingham (ed.) *Reading Audiences: Young People and the Media* Manchester: Manchester University Press

Buckingham, D. (1996) *Moving Images: Understanding Children's Emotional Responses to Television* Manchester: Manchester University Press

Buckingham, D. (ed.) (1988) *Teaching Popular Culture* London: UCL Press

Buckingham, D. (2000a) *After the Death of Childhood: Growing Up in the Age of Electronic Media* Cambridge: Polity

Buckingham, D. (2000b) *The Making of Citizens: Young People, News and Politics* London: UCL Press

Buckingham, D. (2002a) 'Child-centred television? *Teletubbies* and the educational imperative' in D. Buckingham (ed.) *Small Screens: Television for Children* Leicester: Leicester University Press

Buckingham, D. (2002b) 'Introduction: the child and the screen', in D. Buckingham (ed.) *Small Screens: Television for Children* Leicester: Leicester University Press

Buckingham, D. (2003) *Media Education: Learning, Literacy and Contemporary Culture* Cambridge: Polity

Buckingham, D. (2007) *Beyond Technology: Children's Learning in the Age of Digital Culture* Cambridge: Polity

Buckingham, D. (2008a) 'Children and media: a Cultural Studies approach', in K. Drotner and S. Livingstone (eds.) *Handbook of Children, Media and Culture* London: Sage

Buckingham, D. (2008b) 'Introducing identity', in D. Buckingham (ed.) *Youth, Identity and Digital Media* Cambridge, MA: MIT Press

Buckingham, D. (2009a) 'The appliance of science: the role of research in the making of regulatory policy on children and food advertising in the UK', *International Journal of Cultural Policy* 15(2): 201–15

Buckingham, D. (2009b) 'Beyond the competent consumer: the role of media literacy in the making of regulatory policy on children and food advertising in the UK', *International Journal of Cultural Policy* 15(2): 217–30

Buckingham, D. et al. (2009) *The Impact of the Commercial World on Children's Wellbeing: Report of an Independent Assessment* London: Department of Children, Schools and Families and Department of Culture, Media and Sport

Buckingham, D. and Bragg, S. (2004) *Young People, Sex and the Media: The Facts of Life?* London: Palgrave

Buckingham, D. and Bragg, S. (2005) 'Opting into (and out of) childhood: young people, sex and the media', in J. Qvortrup (ed.) *Studies in Modern Childhood: Society, Agency and Culture* London: Sage

Buckingham, D., Bragg, S., Russell, R. and Willett, R. (2010) *Sexualised Goods Aimed at Children* Research report, Edinburgh: Scottish Parliament www.scottish.parliament.uk/s3/committees/equal/reports-10/eor10-02.htm

Buckingham, D., Davies, H., Jones, K. and Kelley, P. (1999) *Children's Television in Britain: History, Discourse and Policy* London: British Film Institute

Buckingham, D. and Scanlon, M. (2003) *Education, Entertainment and Learning in the Home* Buckingham: Open University Press

Buckingham, D. and Scanlon, M. (2005) 'Selling learning: towards a political economy of edutainment media', *Media, Culture and Society* 27(1): 53–68

Buckingham, D., Scanlon, M. and Sefton-Green, J. (2001) 'Selling the digital dream: marketing educational technologies to teachers and parents', in A. Loveless and V. Ellis (eds.) *Subject to Change: Literacy and New Technologies* London: Routledge

Buckingham, D. and Sefton-Green, J. (2003) 'Gotta catch 'em all: structure, agency and pedagogy in children's media culture', *Media, Culture and Society* 25(3): 379–99

Buckingham, D., Whiteman, N., Willett, R. and Burn, A. (2007) *The Impact of the Media on Children and Young People* (review of the literature prepared for the DCSF Byron Review) www.dcsf.gov.uk/byronreview/ (Annex G)

Buijzen, M. (2007) 'Reducing children's susceptibility to commercials: mechanisms of factual and evaluative advertising interventions', *Media Psychology* 9(2): 411–30

Buijzen, M. (2009) 'The effectiveness of parental communication in modifying the relation between food advertising and children's consumption behaviour', *British Journal of Developmental Psychology* 27: 105–21

Buijzen, M. and Mens, C. (2007) 'Adult mediation of television advertising effects: a comparison of factual, evaluative and combined strategies', *Journal of Children and Media* 1(2): 177–91

Buijzen, M. and Valkenburg, P. (2003) 'The unintended effects of television advertising: a parent–child survey', *Communication Research* 30(5): 483–503

Buijzen, M. and Valkenburg, P. (2005) 'Parental mediation of undesired advertising effects', *Journal of Broadcasting and Electronic Media* 49(2): 153–65

Burroughs, J. E. and Rindfleisch, A. (2002) 'Materialism and well-being: a conflicting values perspective', *Journal of Consumer Research* 29: 348–70

Butler, J. (1990) *Gender Trouble* London: Routledge

Calvert, S. (2003) 'The future faces of selling to children', in E. Palmer and B. Young (eds.) *The Faces of Televisual Media: Teaching, Violence, Selling to Children* 2nd edition, Mahwah, NJ: Erlbaum

Campbell, C. (1987) *The Romantic Ethic and the Spirit of Modern Consumerism* Oxford: Blackwell

Campos, P. (2004) *The Obesity Myth: Why America's Obsession with Weight is Hazardous to Your Health* New York: Gotham

Carey, J. (1992) *The Intellectuals and the Masses* London: Faber

Childwise (2009) *Childwise Monitor Survey Report 2008–2009* Norwich: Childwise

Chin, E. (2001) *Purchasing Power: Black Kids and American Consumer Culture* Minneapolis: University of Minnesota Press

Chitty, C. (1997) 'Choice, diversity and equity in secondary schooling', *Oxford Review of Education* 23(1): 45–62

Chubb, J. E. and Moe, T. M. (1990) *Politics, Markets and America's Schools* Washington, DC: Brookings Institute

Chung, G. and Grimes, S. (2005) 'Data mining the kids: surveillance and market research strategies in children's online games', *Canadian Journal of Communication* 30: 527–48

Clark, E. (2007) *The Real Toy Story: Inside the Ruthless Battle for Britain's Youngest Consumers* London: Black Swan

Cohen, L. (2003) *A Consumers' Republic: The Politics of Mass Consumption in Postwar America* New York: Vintage

Cohen, S. (2002) *Folk Devils and Moral Panics* 3rd edition, London: Routledge

Collins, C. and Janning, M. (2010) 'The stuff at mom's house and the stuff at dad's house: the material consumption of divorce for adolescents', in D. Buckingham and V. Tingstad (eds.) *Childhood and Consumer Culture* London: Palgrave Macmillan

Collishaw, S., Maughan, B., Goodman, R. and Pickles, A. (2004) 'Time trends in adolescent mental health', *Journal of Child Psychology and Psychiatry* 45: 1350–62

Compass (2006) *The Commercialisation of Childhood* London: Compass www. compassonline.org.uk/publications/

Cook, D. T. (2000) 'The other "child study": figuring children as consumers in market research, 1910s–1990s', *Sociological Quarterly* 41(3): 487–507

Cook, D. T. (2004) *The Commodification of Childhood: The Children's Clothing Industry and the Rise of the Child Consumer* Durham, NC: Duke University Press

Cook, D. T. (2008) '"The missing child in consumption theory', *Journal of Consumer Culture* 8(2): 219–43

Cook, D. T. (2009a) 'Children's subjectivities and commercial meaning: the delicate battle mothers wage when feeding their children', in A. James, A. T. Kjørholt and V. Tingstad (eds.) *Children, Food and Identity in Everyday Life* London: Palgrave

Cook, D. T. (2009b) 'Semantic provisioning of children's food: commerce, care and maternal practice', *Childhood* 16(3): 317–34

Cook, D. T. (2010) 'Commercial enculturation: moving beyond consumer socialisation', in D. Buckingham and V. Tingstad (eds.) *Childhood and Consumer Culture* London: Palgrave Macmillan

Cook, D. T. and Kaiser, S. (2004) 'Betwixt and be tween: age ambiguity and the sexualization of the female consuming subject', *Journal of Consumer Culture* 4(2): 203–27

Cooper, H. (2000) 'Fleecing kids', *Guardian* 10 June

Corrigan, P. (1997) *The Sociology of Consumption* London: Sage

Corsaro, W. A. (1997) *The Sociology of Childhood* Thousand Oaks, CA: Pine Forge Press

Costello, E. J., Erkanli, A. and Angold, A. (2006) 'Is there an epidemic of child or adolescent depression?' *Journal of Child Psychology and Psychiatry* 47(12): 1263–71

Cowling, J. and Lee, K. (2002) *They Have Been Watching: Children's TV 1955–2002* London: Institute for Public Policy Research

Craik, J. (2009) *Fashion: The Key Concepts* Oxford: Berg

Crewe, L. and Collins, P. (2006) 'Commodifying children: fashion, space, and the production of the profitable child', *Environment and Planning A* 38: 7–24

Crisell, A. (2002) *An Introductory History of British Broadcasting* London: Routledge

Croghan, R., Griffin, C., Hunter, J. and Phoenix, A. (2006) 'Style failure: consumption, identity and social exclusion', *Journal of Youth Studies* 9(4): 463–78

Cross, G. (1997) *Kids' Stuff: Toys and the Changing World of American Childhood* Cambridge, MA: Harvard University Press

Cross, G. (2004) *The Cute and the Cool: Wondrous Innocence and Modern American Children's Culture* New York: Oxford University Press

Cross, G. (2008) *Men to Boys: The Making of Modern Immaturity* New York: Columbia University Press

Cross, G. (2010) 'Children and teens as valves of adult desires', in D. Buckingham and V. Tingstad (eds.) *Childhood and Consumer Culture* London: Palgrave Macmillan

Cuban, L. (2004) *The Blackboard and the Bottom Line: Why Schools Can't Be Businesses* Cambridge, MA: Harvard University Press

Cunningham, H. (2006) *The Invention of Childhood* London: BBC Books

Curran, J. and Seaton, J. (2009) *Power Without Responsibility: Press, Broadcasting and the Internet in Britain* 7th edition, London: Routledge

Davies, H., Buckingham, D. and Kelley, P. (2000) 'In the worst possible taste: children, television and cultural value', *European Journal of Cultural Studies* 3(1): 5–25

Davies, M. and Corbett, B. (1997) *The Provision of Children's Television in Britain* London: Broadcasting Standards Commission

Davis, F. (1992) *Fashion, Culture and Identity* Chicago: University of Chicago Press

Davis, G. and Dickinson, K. (eds.) (2004) *Teen Television: Genre, Culture and Identity* London: British Film Institute

DCSF (Department of Children, Schools and Families) (2007) *The Wellbeing of Children and Young People in the UK: A Review of Available Evidence* London: DCSF

de Block, L. and Buckingham, D. (2007) *Global Children, Global Media: Migration, Media and Childhood* Basingstoke: Palgrave

de Certeau, M. (1984) *The Practice of Everyday Life* Berkeley: University of California Press de Cordova, R. (1994) 'The Mickey in Macy's window: childhood, consumerism and Disney', in E. Smoodin (ed.) *Disney Discourse* London, British Film Institute

de Kervenoael, R., Aykac, D. Selcen O., Hallsworth, A. and Canning, C. (2008) *Capturing Loyalty across Garment Ranges: The Case of Supermarket Children's Clothing in the UK* http://selcen.org/personal/articles/Eirass08_KervenoaelAykacHallsworthCanning.pdf

de Vaney, A. (ed.) (1994) *Watching Channel One: The Convergence of Students, Technology and Private Business* Albany, NY: SUNY Press

de Vault, M. (1991) *Feeding the Family: The Social Organization of Caring as Gendered Work* Chicago: University of Chicago Press

del Vecchio, G. (1997) *Creating Ever-Cool* Louisiana: Pelican

Denisoff, D. (ed.) (2008) *The Nineteenth Century Child and Consumer Culture* Aldershot: Ashgate

Department of Health (2004) *Choosing Health* London: Department of Health

Department of Health (2008) *Changes in Food and Drink Advertising and Promotion to Children* London: DoH

Dickinson, R. (2000) 'Food and eating on television: impacts and influences', *Nutrition & Food Science* 30(1): 24–9

Douglas, M. and Isherwood, B. (1979) *The World of Goods: Towards an Anthropology of Consumption* London: Allen Lane

Dover, C. (2007) 'Everyday talk: investigating media consumption and identity amongst schoolchildren', *Participations* 4(1) www.participations.org

Dryden, C., Metcalfe, A., Owen, J. and Shipton, G. (2009) 'Picturing the lunchbox: children drawing and talking about "dream" and "nightmare" lunchboxes in the primary school setting', in A. James, A. T. Kjørholt and V. Tingstad (eds.) *Children, Food and Identity in Everyday Life* London: Palgrave

Du Gay, P., Hall, S., Janes, L., et al. (1997) *Doing Cultural Studies: The Story of the Sony Walkman* London: Sage

Duits, L. and van Zoonen, L. (2006) 'Headscarves and porno-chic: disciplining girls' bodies in the European multicultural society', *European Journal of Women's Studies* 13(2): 103–17

Duits, L. and van Zoonen, L. (2007) 'Who's afraid of female agency? A rejoinder to Gill', *European Journal of Women's Studies* 14(2): 161–70

Durham, M. G. (2009) *The Lolita Effect: The Media Sexualisation of Young Girls and What You Can Do About It* New York: Overlook

Edwards, T. (2000) *Contradictions of Consumption* London: Sage

Egan, R. D. and Hawkes, G. L. (2007) 'Producing the prurient through the pedagogy of purity: childhood sexuality and the social purity movement', *Journal of Historical Sociology* 20(4): 443–61

Egan, R. D. and Hawkes, G. L. (2008) 'Endangered girls and incendiary objects: unpacking the discourse on sexualisation', *Sexuality and Culture* 12: 291–311

Egan, R. D. and Hawkes, G. L. (2010) *Theorizing the Sexual Child in Modernity* London: Palgrave Macmillan

Ehrenreich, B. (1990) *Fear of Falling: The Inner Life of the Middle Class* New York: Harper Perennial

Ekstrom, K. (2006) 'Consumer socialization revisited', in R. W. Belk (ed.) *Research in Consumer Behavior*, vol. X Oxford: Elsevier

Ekstrom, K. (2007) 'Parental consumer learning or "keeping up with the children"', *Journal of Consumer Behaviour* 6: 203–17

Elliott, R. and Leonard, C. (2004) 'Peer pressure and poverty: exploring fashion brands and consumption symbolism among the children of the "British poor"', *Journal of Consumer Behaviour* 3(4): 347–59

Engelhardt, T. (1986) 'Children's television: the shortcake strategy', in T. Gitlin (ed.), *Watching Television* New York: Pantheon

Erikson, E. (1968) *Identity: Youth and Crisis* New York: Norton

ESRC (Economic and Social Research Council) (2006) *Changing Household and Family Structures and Complex Living Arrangements* Swindon: ESRC

Evans, J. and Chandler, J. (2006) 'To buy or not to buy: family dynamics and children's consumption', *Sociological Research Online* 11(2) www.socresonline.org.uk/11/2/evans.html

Evans, J., Davies, B. and Rich, E. (2008a) 'The class and cultural functions of obesity discourse: our latter day child saving movement', *International Studies in Sociology of Education* 18(2): 117–32

Evans, J., Rich, E., Davies, B. and Allwood, R. (2008b) *Education, Disordered Eating and Obesity Discourse: Fat Fabrications* London: Routledge

Eveleth, P. B. (1986) 'Timing of menarche: secular trends and population difference', in J. B. Lancaster and B. A. Hamburg (eds.) *School-age Pregnancy and Parenthood* New York: Aldine de Gruyter

Facer, K., Furlong, J., Furlong, R. and Sutherland, R. (2003) *Screenplay: Children and Computing in the Home* London: Routledge

Featherstone, M. (1991) *Consumer Culture and Postmodernism* London: Sage

Fiedler, A., Gardner, W., Nairn, A. and Pitt, J. (2007) *Fair Game? Assessing Commercial Activity on Children's Favourite Websites and Online Environments* London: National Consumer Council

Fine, B. (2002) *The World of Consumption: The Material and Cultural Revisited* London: Routledge

Fine, C. and Nairn, A. (2008) 'Who's messing with my mind? The implication of dual process models for the ethics of advertising to children', *International Journal of Advertising* 27(3): 447–70

Fiske, J. (1987) *Television Culture* London: Methuen

Fiske, J. (1990) *Understanding Popular Culture* London: Unwin Hyman

Fitz, J. and Hafid, T. (2007) 'Perspectives on the privatization of public schooling' *Educational Policy* 21(1): 273–96

Fletcher, W. (2003) 'Tween power? You're kidding' *Times Higher Educational Supplement* 2 May, www.timeshighereducation.co.uk/story.asp?storyCode=1 76377&sectioncode=9

Foresight (2007) *Tackling Obesities – Future Choices: Project Report* London: Government Office for Science

Foucault, M. (1978) *The History of Sexuality*, vol. I, Harmondsworth: Penguin

France, A., Meredith, J. and Murdock, G. (2009) *Children and Marketing: Literature Review*, Appendix H of the DCSF/DCMS Report *The Impact of the Commercial World on Children's Wellbeing* London: DCSF

Freedman, J. (2002) *Media Violence and its Effect on Aggression: Assessing the Scientific Evidence* Toronto: University of Toronto Press

Frosh, S., Phoenix, A. and Pattman, R. (2002) *Young Masculinities: Understanding Boys in Contemporary Society* Basingstoke: Palgrave

Furedi, F. (2008) *Paranoid Parenting* London: Continuum

Gabriel, Y. and Lang, T. (2006) *The Unmanageable Consumer* 2nd edition, London: Sage

Galbraith, J. K. (1958) *The Affluent Society* Boston: Houghton Mifflin

Gard, D. and Wright, J. (2005) *The Obesity Epidemic: Science, Morality and Ideology* London: Routledge

Giacquinta, J. B., Bauer, J. and Levin, J. E. (1993) *Beyond Technology's Promise: An Examination of Children's Educational Computing at Home* Cambridge: Cambridge University Press

Giddens, A. (1984) *The Constitution of Society* Cambridge: Polity

Giddens, A. (1991) *Modernity and Self-Identity* Cambridge: Polity

Giddens, A. (1992) *The Transformation of Intimacy: Sexuality, Love and Eroticism in Modern Societies* Cambridge: Polity

Gill, R. C. (2007) 'Critical respect: the difficulties and dilemmas of agency and "choice" for feminism', *European Journal of Women's Studies* 14(1): 69–80

Gill, R. C. (2008) 'Empowerment/agency: figuring female sexual agency in contemporary advertising', *Feminism and Psychology* 18(1): 35–60

Goldberg, M. E., Gorn, G. J., Peracchio, L. A. and Bamossy, G. (2003) 'Understanding materialism among youth', *Journal of Consumer Psychology* 13: 278–88

Gordon, D., Levitas, R. and Pantazis, C. (eds.) (2006) *Poverty and Social Exclusion in Britain: The Millennium Survey* Bristol: Policy Press

Gram, M. (2010) 'Children's roles in family supermarket shopping', paper presented at Child and Teen Consumption Conference, Linkoping, Sweden, June

Greenfield, P. M., Yut, E., Chung, M., et al. (1990) 'The program-length commercial: a study of the effects of television/toy tie-ins on imaginative play', *Psychology and Marketing* 7(4): 237–55

Grimes, S. and Shade, L. R. (2005) 'Neopian economics of play: children's cyberpets and online communities as immersive advertising in Neopets.com', *International Journal of Media and Cultural Politics* 1(2): 181–98

Guldberg, H. (2008) *Reclaiming Childhood: Freedom and Play in an Age of Fear* London: Routledge

Gunter, B. and Furnham, A. (1998) *Children as Consumers* London: Routledge

Gunter, B., Oates, C. and Blades, M. (2005) *Advertising to Children on TV: Context, Impact and Regulation* London: Routledge

Halifax Pocket Money Survey (2009) News report 11 December http://news.bbc.co.uk/1/hi/uk/8409323.stm

Hall, S. (1992) 'The question of cultural identity', in S. Hall, D. Held and A. McGrew (eds.) *Modernity and its Futures* Cambridge: Polity

Hall, S. and Jacques, M. (eds.) (1989) *New Times: The Changing Face of Politics in the 1990s* London: Lawrence and Wishart

Harris, A. (2004a) *Future Girl: Young Women in the Twenty First Century* New York: Routledge

Harris, A. (ed.) (2004b) *All About the Girl: Culture, Power and Identity* London: Routledge

Hartley, D. (2008) 'Education, markets and the pedagogy of personalisation', *British Journal of Educational Studies* 56(4): 365–81

Harty, S. (1979) *Hucksters in the Classroom: A Review of Industry Propaganda in Schools* Washington, DC: Center for the Study of Responsive Law

Hastings, G., Stead, M., McDermott, L., et al. (2003) *Review of Research on the Effects of Food Promotion to Children* Glasgow: Centre for Social Marketing, University of Strathclyde

Hawkes, G. L. and Egan, R. D. (2008) 'Girls, sexuality and the strange carnalities of advertisements', *Australian Feminist Studies* 23(57): 307–22

Hayward, K. and Yar, M. (2006) 'The "chav" phenomenon: consumption, media and the construction of a new underclass', *Crime, Media, Culture* 2(1): 9–28

Hendershot, H. (1998) *Saturday Morning Censors: Television Regulation before the V-Chip* Durham, NC: Duke University Press

Hendershot, H. (2004) 'Introduction', in H. Hendershot (ed.) *Nickelodeon Nation: The History, Politics and Economics of America's Only TV Channel for Kids* New York: New York University Press

Hesmondhalgh, D. (2007) *The Cultural Industries* 2nd edition, London: Sage

Higonnet, A. (1998) *Pictures of Innocence: The History and Crisis of Ideal Childhood* London: Thames and Hudson

Hilgartner, S. and Bosk, C. (1988) 'The rise and fall of social problems: a public arenas model', *American Journal of Sociology* 94(1): 53–78

Hjarvard, S. (2004) 'From bricks to bytes: the mediatization of a global toy industry', in I. Bjondeberg and P. Golding (eds.) *European Culture and the Media* Bristol: Intellect

Hollows, J. (2003) 'Oliver's twist: leisure, labour and domestic masculinity in *The Naked Chef*', *International Journal of Cultural Studies* 6(2): 229–48

Home Office (2010) *Sexualisation of Young People Review* London: Home Office www.homeoffice.gov.uk/documents/Sexualisation-young-people

Howe, C. (2010) *Peer Groups and Children's Development: Psychological and Educational Perspectives* Chichester: Wiley-Blackwell

Husen, M. O. (2009) 'Nature, functionality and aesthetics: advertisements and notions of a "good" childhood', unpublished paper, Norwegian Centre for Child Research, NTNU Trondheim

Ingelhart, R. (1981) 'Post-materialism in an environment of insecurity', *American Political Science Review* 75(4): 880–900

Ingelhart, R. and Abramson, P. R. (1999) 'Measuring postmaterialism', *American Political Science Review* 93(3): 665–77

Ireson, J. (2004) 'Private tutoring: how prevalent and effective is it?' *London Review of Education* 2(2): 109–22

Ito, M. (2009) *Engineering Play: A Cultural History of Children's Software* Cambridge, MA: MIT Press

Ito, M., Baumer, S., Bittanti, M., et al. (2010) *Hanging Out, Messing Around and Geeking Out* Cambridge, MA: MIT Press

Jackson, S. (1982) *Childhood and Sexuality* Oxford: Blackwell

Jacobson, L. (2004) *Raising Consumers: Children and the American Mass Market in the Early Twentieth Century* New York: Columbia University Press

James, A. (1982) 'Confections, concoctions and conceptions', in B. Waites, T. Bennett and G. Martin (eds.) *Popular Culture: Past and Present* London: Croom Helm / Open University Press

James, A. (1993) *Childhood Identities* Edinburgh: Edinburgh University Press

James, A., Curtis, P. and Ellis, K. (2009) 'Negotiating family, negotiating food: children ad family participants?', in A. James, A. T. Kjørholt and V. Tingstad (eds.) *Children, Food and Identity in Everyday Life* London: Palgrave

James, A., Jenks, C. and Prout, A. (1998) *Theorizing Childhood* Cambridge: Polity

James, A. and Prout, A. (eds.) (1990) *Constructing and Reconstructing Childhood: Contemporary Issues in the Sociological Study of Childhood* London: Falmer

James, O. (2007) *Affluenza* London: Vermilion

James, O. (2010) *How Not To F*** Them Up* London: Vermilion

Jenkins, H. (2004) 'Interview with Geraldine Laybourne', in H. Hendershot (ed.) *Nickelodeon Nation: The History, Politics and Economics of America's Only TV Channel for Kids* New York: New York University Press

Jenkins, P. (1992) *Intimate Enemies: Moral Panics in Contemporary Great Britain* New York: Aldine de Gruyter

Jenkins, R. (2004) *Social Identity* 2nd edition, London: Routledge

Johansson, B. (2010) 'Subjectivities of the child consumer: beings and becomings', in D. Buckingham and V. Tingstad (eds.) *Childhood and Consumer Culture* London: Palgrave Macmillan

John, D. R. (1999) 'Consumer socialization of children: a retrospective look at twenty-five years of research', *Journal of Consumer Research* 26(3): 183–213

Johnson, R. (1985/6) 'What is Cultural Studies anyway?' *Social Text* 16: 38–80; republished in J. Storey (ed.) (1996) *What is Cultural Studies? A Reader* London: Edward Arnold

Jordanova, L. (1989) 'Children in history: concepts of nature and society', in G. Scarre (ed.) *Children, Parents and Politics* Cambridge: Cambridge University Press

Julier, A. (2008) 'The political economy of obesity: the fat pay all', in C. Counihan and P. van Esterik (eds.) *Food and Culture: A Reader* London: Routledge

Kaplowitz, P. B., Slora, E., Wasserman, R. C., Pedlow, S. E. and Herman-Giddens, M. E. (2001) 'Early onset of puberty in girls: relation to increased body mass index and race', *Pediatrics* 108(2): 347–53

Kasser, T., Ryan, R. M., Couchman, C. E. and Sheldon, K. M. (2004) 'Materialistic values: Their causes and consequences', in T. Kasser and A. D. Kanner (eds.) *Psychology and Consumer Culture: The Struggle for a Good Life in a Materialistic World* Washington, DC: American Psychological Association

Katz, C. (2004) *Growing Up Global: Economic Restructuring and Children's Everyday Lives* Minneapolis: University of Minnesota Press

Kaveney, R. (2006) *Teen Dreams: Reading Teen Film and Television from 'Heathers' to 'Veronica Mars'* London: I. B.Tauris

Kehily, M. J. (1999) 'More sugar? Teenage magazines, gender displays and sexual learning', *European Journal of Cultural Studies* 2(1): 65–89

Kehily, M. J. and Montgomery, H. (2002) 'Innocence and experience: a historical approach to childhood sexuality', in M. Woodhead and H. Montgomery (eds.) *Understanding Childhood: An Interdisciplinary Approach* Chichester: Wiley

Kelley, P., Buckingham, D. and Davies, H. (1999) 'Talking dirty: children, sexual knowledge and television', *Childhood* 6(2): 221–42

Kenway, J. and Bullen, E. (2001) *Consuming Children: Education–Entertainment–Advertising* Buckingham: Open University Press

Kerawalla, L. and Crook, C. (2005) 'From promises to practices: the fate of educational software in the home', *Technology, Pedagogy and Education* 14(1): 107–25

Kiernan, K., Lewis, J. and Land, H. (1998) *Lone Motherhood in Twentieth-Century Britain* Oxford: Oxford University Press

Kincaid, J. (1992) *Child Loving: The Erotic Child and Victorian Culture* London: Routledge

Kincaid, J. (1998) *The Culture of Child Molesting* Durham, NC: Duke University Press

Kinder, M. (1991) *Playing with Power in Movies, Television and Video Games: From Muppet Babies to Teenage Mutant Ninja Turtles* Berkeley: University of California Press

Klein, N. (2001) *No Logo* London: Flamingo

Kline, S. (1993) *Out of the Garden: Toys and Children's Culture in the Age of TV Marketing* London: Verso

Kooistra, L. J. (2008) '*Home Thoughts* and *Home Scenes*: Packaging Middle-Class Childhood for Christmas Consumption', in D. Denisoff (ed.) *The Nineteenth-Century Child and Consumer Culture* Aldershot: Ashgate

Korsvold, T. (2010) 'Proper toys for proper children: a case study of the Norwegian company A/S Riktige Leker (Proper Toys)', in D. Buckingham and V. Tingstad (eds.) *Childhood and Consumer Culture* London: Palgrave Macmillan

Korsvold, T. (in press) 'Revisiting constructions of children and youths in marketing advertisements: an historical and empirical study of the company Helle Hansen', submitted to *Young: Journal of Youth Research*

Kunkel, D. (1988) 'From a raised eyebrow to a turned back: the FCC and children's product-related programming', *Journal of Communication* 38(4): 90–108

Lamb, S. and Brown, L. M. (2006) *Packaging Girlhood: Rescuing Our Daughters from Marketers' Schemes* New York: St Martins Griffin

Lang, T. and Heasman, M. (2004) *Food Wars: The Global Battle for Mouths, Minds and Markets* London: Earthscan

Lareau, A. (2003) *Unequal Childhoods: Class, Race and Family Life* Berkeley: University of California Press

Larson, R., Branscomb, K. and Wiley, A. (2006) 'Forms and functions of family mealtimes: multidisciplinary perspectives', *New Directions of Child and Adolescent Development* 111: 1–15

Lash, S. and Lury, C. (2007) *Global Culture Industry: The Mediation of Things* Cambridge: Polity

Lauder, H. and Hughes, D. (eds.) (1999) *Trading in Futures: Why Markets in Education Don't Work* Buckingham: Open University Press

Lawlor, M.-A. and Prothero, A. (2003) 'Children's understanding of television advertising intent', *Journal of Marketing Management* 19(3–4): 411–31

Layard, R. (2005) *Happiness: Lessons from a New Science* London: Penguin

Layard, R. and Dunn, J. (2009) *A Good Childhood: Searching for Values in a Competitive Age* London: Penguin

Laybourne, G. (1993) 'The Nickelodeon experience', in G. Berry and J. Asamen (eds.) *Children and Television: Images in a Changing Sociocultural World* Beverly Hills: Sage

Lee, N. (2001) *Childhood and Society: Growing Up in an Age of Uncertainty* Buckingham: Open University Press

Lemish, D. and Bloch, L.-R. (2004) 'Pokémon in Israel', in J. Tobin (ed.) *Pikachu's Global Adventure: The Rise and Fall of Pokémon* Durham, NC: Duke University Press

Levin, D. and Kilbourne, J. (2008) *So Sexy So Soon: The New Sexualised Childhood and What Parents Can Do to Protect Their Kids* New York: Ballantine

Levine, J. (2002) *Harmful to Minors: The Perils of Protecting Children from Sex* Minneapolis and London: University of Minnesota Press

Levy, A. (2006) *Female Chauvinist Pigs: Women and the Rise of Raunch Culture* London: Pocket Books

Lindstrom, M. and Seybold, P. (2003) *Brandchild* London: Kogan Page

Linn, S. (2004) *Consuming Kids: The Hostile Takeover of Childhood* New York: New Press

Liverpool Victoria Friendly Society (2010) 'The cost of raising a child tops £200,000', press release, 23 February www.lv.com/media_centre/press_releases/

Livingstone, S. (2004) *A Commentary on the Research Evidence Regarding the Effects of Food Promotion on Children* London: London School of Economics

Livingstone, S. (2006a) 'Children's privacy online', in R. Kraut, M. Brynin and S. Kiesler (eds.) *Computers, Phones and the Internet* New York: Oxford University Press

Livingstone, S. (2006b) *New Research on Advertising Foods to Children: An Updated Review of the Literature* Annex 9 of Ofcom *Television Advertising of Food and Drink Products to Children* London: Ofcom

Livingstone, S. and Bovill, M. (1999) *Young People, New Media* London: London School of Economics and Political Science

Livingstone, S. and Helsper, E. (2004) *Advertising Foods to Children: Understanding Promotion in the Context of Children's Daily Lives* London: London School of Economics

Livingstone, S. and Helsper, E. (2006) 'Does advertising literacy mediate the effects of advertising on children? A critical examination of two linked research literatures in relation to obesity and food choice', *Journal of Communication* 56: 560–84

Lodziak, C. (2002) *The Myth of Consumerism* London: Pluto

Loseke, D. R. (2003) *Thinking about Social Problems: An Introduction to Constructionist Perspectives* New Brunswick: Aldine Transaction

Luke, C. (1989) *Pedagogy, Printing and Protestantism: The Discourse on Childhood* Albany, NY: SUNY Press

Lukose, R. A. (2009) *Liberalization's Children: Gender, Youth and Consumer Citizenship in Globalizing India* Durham, NC: Duke University Press

Lumby, C. and Albury, K. (2008) 'Submission to the Senate Standing Committee on Environment, Communication and the Arts Inquiry into the Sexualisation of Children in the Contemporary Media Environment', University of New South Wales

Lurie, A. (1983) *The Language of Clothes* London: Hamlyn

Lurie, A. (1990) *Don't Tell the Grown-Ups: Subversive Children's Literature* Chicago: Little, Brown and Company

Lury, C. (1996) *Consumer Culture* Cambridge: Polity

Lury, C. (2004) *Brands: The Logos of the Global Economy* London: Routledge

Luthar, S. S. (2003) 'The culture of affluence: psychological costs of material wealth', *Child Development* 74(6): 1581–93

Luthar, S. S. and Latendresse, S. J. (2005) 'Children of the affluent: challenges to well-being', *Current Directions in Psychological Science* 14(1): 49–53

Mackay, H. (ed.) (1997) *Consumption and Everyday Life* London: Sage

Marshall, D., O'Donohoe, S. and Kline, S. (2007) 'Families, food and pester power: beyond the blame game?' *Journal of Consumer Behavior* 6: 164–81

Martens, L. (2005) 'Safety, safety, safety for small fry: the conjoining of children and danger in commercial communities of parenthood', unpublished conference paper presented at the Childhoods 2005 conference, Oslo, June

Martens, L, Southerton, D. and Scott, S. (2004) 'Bringing children (and parents) into the sociology of consumption', *Journal of Consumer Culture* 4(2): 155–82

Mayo, E. and Nairn, A. (2009) *Consumer Kids: How Big Business is Grooming Our Children for Profit* London: Constable

McCracken, G. (1988) *Culture and Consumption: New Approaches to the Symbolic Character of Consumer Goods and Activities* Bloomington: Indiana University Press

McGinnis, J. M., Appleton Gootman, J. and Kraak, V. I. (eds.) (2006) *Food Marketing to Children: Threat or Opportunity?* Washington, DC: National Academies Press

McGray, D. (2002) 'Japan's gross national cool', *Foreign Policy* (May–June)

McGuigan, J. (1998) 'Cultural populism revisited', in M. Ferguson and P. Golding (eds.) *Cultural Studies in Question* London: Sage

McKechnie, J., Hobbs, S. and Anderson, S. (2004) *Child Employment in Britain* Glasgow: University of Paisley

McKendrick, J. H., Bradford, M. G. and Fielder, A. V. (2000) 'Kid customer? Commercialization of playspace and the commodification of childhood' *Childhood* 7(3): 295–314

McKendrick, N., Brewer, J. and Plumb, J. H. (1982) *The Birth of a Consumer Society: The Commercialization of Eighteenth-Century England* London: Europa Publications

McNair, B. (2002) *Striptease Culture: Sex, Media and the Democratisation of Desire* London: Routledge

McNeal, J. U. (1992) *Kids as Customers: A Handbook of Marketing to Children* New York: Lexington Books

McNeal, J. U. (1999) *The Children's Market: Myths and Realities* New York: Paramount

McNeal, J. U. (2007) *On Becoming a Consumer: Development of Consumer Behavior Patterns in Childhood* Burlington, MA: Butterworth-Heinemann

McNeal, J. U. and Yeh, C.-H. (2003) 'The consumer behaviour of Chinese children, 1995–2002', *Journal of Consumer Marketing* 20(6): 542–54

Melody, W. (1973) *Children's Television: The Economics of Exploitation* New Haven: Yale University Press

Mennell, S. (1985) *All Manners of Food: Eating and Taste in England and France from the Middle Ages to the Present* Oxford: Blackwell

Middleton, S., Ashworth, K. and Braithwaite, I. (1998) *Small Fortunes: Spending on Children, Childhood and Parental Sacrifice* York: Joseph Rowntree Foundation

Miles, S. (1998) *Consumerism as a Way of Life* London: Sage

Miles, S., Cliff, D. and Burr, V. (1998) 'Fitting in and sticking out: consumption, consumer meanings and the construction of young people's identities', *Journal of Youth Studies* 1(1): 81–91

Miller, D. (1987) *Material Culture and Mass Consumption* Oxford: Blackwell

Miller, D. (1997) 'Consumption and its consequences', in Mackay, H. (ed.) *Consumption and Everyday Life* London: Sage

Miller, D. (1998) *A Theory of Shopping* Cambridge: Polity

Miller, D. (2008) *The Comfort of Things* Cambridge: Polity

Millwood Hargrave, A. and Livingstone, S. (2006) *Harm and Offence in Media Content: A Review of the Evidence* Bristol: Intellect

Milner, M. (2004) *Freaks, Geeks and Cool Kids: American Teenagers, Schools, and the Culture of Consumption* New York: Routledge

Mizen, P., Bolton, A. and Pole, C. (1999) 'School age workers: the paid employment of children in Britain', *Work, Employment and Society* 13: 423–38

Molnar, A. (2005) *School Commercialism: From Democratic Ideal to Market Commodity* New York: Routledge

Molnar, A. and Boninger, F. (2007) *Adrift: Schools in a Total Marketing Environment* Tempe, AZ: Arizona State University http://epsl.asu.edu/ceru/CERU_2007_Annual_Report.htm

Monaghan, L. (2007) *Men and the War on Obesity* London: Routledge

Montgomery, K. (2007) *Generation Digital* Cambridge, MA: MIT Press

Montgomery, K. and Chester, J. (2007) 'Food advertising to children in the new digital marketing ecosystem', in K. Ekstrom and B. Tufte (eds.) *Children, Media and Consumption: On the Front Edge* Goteborg, Sweden: Nordicom

Montgomery, K. and Chester, J. (2009) 'Interactive food and beverage marketing: targeting adolescents in the digital age', *Journal of Adolescent Health* 45(3), Suppplement: S18–S29

Morrow, V. and Mayall, B. (2009) 'What is wrong with children's well-being in the UK? Questions of meaning and measurement', *Journal of Social Welfare and Family Law* 31(3): 217–29

Murdock, G. (1990) 'Television and citizenship', in A. Tomlinson (ed.) *Consumption, Identity and Style* London: Routledge

Nadesan, M. H. (2002) 'Engineering the entrepreneurial infant: brain science, infant development toys, and governmentality', *Cultural Studies* 16(3): 401–32

Nairn, A. and Dew, A. (2007) 'Pop-ups, pop-unders, banners and buttons: the ethics of on-line advertising to primary school children', *Journal of Direct, Data and Digital Marketing Practice* 9(1): 30–46

Nairn, A. and Monkgol, D. (2007) 'Children and privacy online', *Journal of Direct, Data and Digital Marketing Practice* 8: 294–308

Nairn, A., Ormrod, J. and Bottomley, P. (2006) *Watching, Wanting and Wellbeing: Exploring the Links* London: National Consumer Council

Nairn, A., Ormrod, J. and Bottomley, P. (2010) ' "Those who have less want more. But does it make them feel bad?" Deprivation, materialism and self-esteem in childhood', in D. Buckingham and V. Tingstad (eds.) *Childhood and Consumer Culture* Basingstoke: Palgrave

Nash, C. (2009) 'The parent–child purchase relationship'. M.Phil. thesis, Dublin Institute of Technology

National Union of Teachers (2007) *Growing Up in a Material World* London: NUT

Nieuwenhuys, O. (1996) 'The paradox of child labour and anthropology' *Annual Review of Anthropology* 25: 237–51

Nixon, H. (1998) 'Fun and games are serious business', in J. Sefton-Green (ed.) *Digital Diversions: Youth Culture in the Age of Multimedia* London: UCL Press

Norgaard, M. K. and Brunso, K. (2010) 'Barriers experienced in the supermarket by parents and children during family food buying', paper presented at Child and Teen Consumption Conference, Linkoping, Sweden, June

Oates, C. (2009) 'Food content in children's UK television programmes', in *Proceedings of the Academy of Marketing Conference*, Leeds: Leeds Metropolitan University

Oates, C., Blades, M. and Gunter, B. (2002) 'Children and television advertising: when do they understand persuasive intent?' *Journal of Consumer Behavior* 1(3): 238–45

Ofcom (2004) *Child Obesity – Food Advertising in Context* London: Ofcom www.ofcom.org.uk/research/tv/reports/food_ads/

Ofcom (2006) 'New restrictions on the television advertising of food and drink products to children' news release, London: Ofcom www.ofcom.org.uk/media/news/2006/11/nr_20061117

Ofcom (2007a) *Final Statement on the Television Advertising of Food and Drink Products to Children* London: Ofcom www.ofcom.org.uk/media/mofaq/bdc/foodadsfaq/

Ofcom. (2007b) *The Future of Children's Television Programming* London: Ofcom

Ofcom (2007c) *The Future of Children's Television Programming: Research Report* London: Ofcom

Ofcom (2008a) *Review of the Effects of the HFSS Advertising Restrictions* London: Ofcom

Ofcom (2008b) *Trends in Advertising Spend across Media* London: Ofcom

Office of Fair Trading (2004) *A Strategy and Framework for Consumer Education* London: OFT

Office of National Statistics (2007) *Families in Focus* London: ONS

Ofsted (Office for Standards in Education) (2007) *Tellus2: Children and Young People Survey* London: Ofsted

Oswell, D. (2002) *Television, Childhood, and the Home* Oxford: Oxford University Press

Quart, A. (2003) *Branded: The Buying and Selling of Teenagers* London: Arrow

Packard, V. (1957) *The Hidden Persuaders* New York: McKay

PACT (2006) 'Children's programming threatened: ad ban threatens investment in children's programming' London: PACT www.pact.co.uk/detail. asp?id=5557

Palmer, E. (1987) *Children in the Cradle of Television* Lexington: Lexington Books

Palmer, S. (2006) *Toxic Childhood: How the Modern World is Damaging Our Children and What We Can Do About It* London: Orion

Palmer, S. (2007) *Detoxing Childhood: What Parents Need to Know to Raise Happy, Successful Children* London: Orion

Parker, J. (2000) *Structuration* Buckingham: Open University Press

Patel, R. (2007) *Stuffed and Starved: From Farm to Fork, the Hidden Battle for the World Food System* London: Portobello

Paterson, M. (2006) *Consumption and Everyday Life* London: Routledge

Phoenix, A. (2009) 'Young consumers', in S. Ding and K. Littleton (eds.) *Children's Personal and Social Development* Chichester: Wiley-Blackwell

Phoenix, A. (2010) '(Ir)resistible consumption: gender, social class and flexible identity projects', keynote presentation at Child and Teen Consumption Conference, Linkoping, Sweden, June

Pilcher, J. (2010) 'What not to wear? Girls, clothing and "showing" the body', *Children and Society* 24(6): 461–70

Pilcher, J., Pole, C. and Boden, S. (2004) 'New consumers? The social and cultural significance of children's fashion consumption', paper presented at Knowing Consumers: Actors, Images and Identities in Modern History Conference, Bielefeld, Germany, 27–28 February www.consume.bbk.ac.uk/research/pole.html

Plumb, J. H. (1982) 'Children and consumption', in N. McKendrick, J. Brewer and J. H. Plumb *The Birth of a Consumer Society: The Commercialization of Eighteenth-Century England* London: Europa Publications

Pole, C., Boden, S., Edwards, T. and Pilcher, J. (2005) 'New consumers: children. Fashion and consumption', End of Award Report, Swindon: Economic and Social Research Council

Pomerantz, S. (2008) *Girls, Style, and School Identities: Dressing the Part* Basingstoke: Palgrave

Postman, N. (1983) *The Disappearance of Childhood* London: W. H. Allen

Potter, J. and Wetherell, M. (1987) *Discourse and Social Psychology* London: Sage

Prentice, A. M. and Jebb, S. A. (1995) 'Obesity in Britain: gluttony or sloth?' *British Medical Journal* 311: 437–9

Pugh, A. G. (2009) *Longing and Belonging: Parents, Children and Consumer Culture* Berkeley: University of California Press

Raine, G. (2007) 'Commercial activities in primary schools: a quantitative study', *Oxford Review of Education* 33(2): 211–31

Rampton, B., Harris, R. and Dover, C. (2002) 'Interaction, media culture and adolescents at school' www.identities.org.uk

Reist, M. T. (2009) *Getting Real: Challenging the Sexualization of Girls* Melbourne: Spinifex Press

Ridge, T. (2002) *Childhood Poverty and Social Exclusion* Bristol: Policy Press

Ringel, P. (2008) 'Reforming the delinquent child consumer: institutional responses to children's consumption from the late nineteenth century to the present', in L. Jacobson (ed.) *Children and Consumer Culture in American Society* Westport, CN: Praeger

Roberts, P. (1994) 'Business sponsorship in schools: a changing climate', in D. Bridges and T. McLaughlin (eds.) *Education and the Market Place* London: Falmer

Rose, C. (2010) *Making, Selling and Wearing Boys' Clothes in Late-Victorian England* Aldershot: Ashgate

Rose, N. (1999) *Governing the Soul* 2nd edition, London: Free Association

Rosen, A. (2003) *The Transformation of British Life, 1950–2000* Manchester: Manchester University Press

Rowland, W. (1983) *The Politics of TV Violence: Policy Uses of Communication Research* Beverly Hills: Sage

Rush, E. and La Nauze, A. (2006) *Corporate Paedophilia: Sexualisation of Children in Australia* Canberra: The Australia Institute

Russell, R. and Tyler, M. (2002) 'Thank heaven for little girls: "girl heaven" and the commercial context of feminine childhood', *Sociology* 36(3): 619–37

Russell, R. and Tyler, M. (2005) 'Branding and bricolage: gender, consumption and transition', *Childhood* 12(2): 221–37

Rysst, M. (2010) '"Hello – we are only in the fifth grade!" Children's rights, inter-generationality and constructions of gender in public debates about childhood', in D. Buckingham and V. Tingstad (eds.) *Childhood and Consumer Culture* Basingstoke: Palgrave

Schee, C. V. (2009) 'Fruit, vegetables, fatness, and Foucault: governing students and their families through school health policy', *Journal of Education Policy* 24(5): 557–74

Schneider, C. (1987) *Children's Television: The Art, The Business and How it Works* Lincolnwood, IL: NTC Business Books

Schor, J. (2004) *Born to Buy: The Commercialized Child and the New Consumer Culture* New York: Scribner

Seiter, E. (1993) *Sold Separately: Parents and Children in Consumer Culture* New Brunswick, NJ: Rutgers University Press

Seiter, E. (1999) *Television and New Media Audiences* Oxford: Oxford University Press

Siegel, D. L., Coffey, T. J. and Livingston, G. (2001) *The Great Tween Buying Machine: Marketing to Today's Tweens* Ithaca, NY: Paramount Market Publishing

Simensky, L. (2004) 'The early days of Nicktoons', in H. Hendershot (ed.) *Nickelodeon Nation: The History, Politics and Economics of America's Only TV Channel for Kids* New York: New York University Press

Skaar, H. (2010) 'Branded selves: how children relate to marketing on a social network site', in D. Buckingham and V. Tingstad (eds.) *Childhood and Consumer Culture* Basingstoke: Palgrave

Skaar, H., Buckingham, D. and Tingstad, V. (2010) 'Marketing on the internet: a new educational challenge', *Media Education Research Journal* 1(2): 13–30

Slater, D. (1997) *Consumer Culture and Modernity* Cambridge: Polity

Slonje, R. and Smith, P. K. (2007) 'Cyberbullying', *Scandinavian Journal of Psychology* 49(2): 147–54

Smith, J. (2010) 'The books that sing: the marketing of children's phonograph records, 1890–1930', in D. Buckingham and V. Tingstad (eds.) *Childhood and Consumer Culture* London: Palgrave Macmillan

Smythe, D. (1981) *Dependency Road: Communications, Capitalism, Consciousness, and Canada* Norwood, NJ: Ablex

Snow, D. and Benford, R. (1988) 'Ideology, frame resistance, and participant mobilization', in B. Klandermans, H. Kriesi and S. Tarrow, S. (eds.) *International Social Movement Research* Greenwich, CT: JAI

Social Issues Research Centre (2005) *Obesity and the Facts* Oxford: SIRC

Social Issues Research Centre (2009a) *Childhood and Family Life: Socio-Demographic Changes* Oxford: SIRC

Social Issues Research Centre (2009b) *The Ecology of Family Life* Oxford: SIRC

Spigel, L. (1992) *Make Room for TV* Chicago: University of Chicago Press

Springhall, J. (1998) *Youth, Popular Culture and Moral Panics* London: Macmillan

Steele, J. R. (1999) 'Teenage sexuality and media practice: factoring in the influences of family, friends and school', *Journal of Sex Research* 36(4): 331–41

Steemers, J. (2010) *Creating Preschool Television: A Story of Commerce, Creativity and Curriculum* Basingstoke: Palgrave

Sternheimer, K. (2010) *Connecting Social Problems and Popular Culture* Boulder, CO: Westview

Sutherland, A. and Thompson, B. (2001) *Kidfluence: Why Kids Today Mean Business* New York: McGraw Hill

Swain, J. (2002) 'The right stuff: fashioning an identity through clothing in a junior school', *Gender in Education* 14(1): 53–69

Swingewood, A. (1977) *The Myth of Mass Culture* London: Macmillan

Thomas, S. G. (2007) *Buy, Buy Baby* London: Harper Collins

Tingstad, V. (2009) 'Discourses on child obesity and TV advertising in the context of the Norwegian welfare state', in A. James, A. T. Kjørholt and V. Tingstad (eds.) *Children, Food and Identity in Everyday Life* London: Palgrave

Tobin, J. (ed.) (2004) *Pikachu's Global Adventure: The Rise and Fall of Pokémon* Durham, NC: Duke University Press

Tooley, J. (1994) 'In defence of markets in educational provision', in D. Bridges and T. McLaughlin (eds.) *Education and the Market Place* London: Falmer

Torell, V. B. (2004) 'Adults and children debating sexy girls' clothes', in H. Brembeck, B. Johansson and J. Kampmann (eds.) *Beyond the Competent Child: Exploring Contemporary Childhoods in the Nordic Welfare Societies* Fredericksberg: Roskilde University Press

Turow, J. (1981) *Entertainment, Education and the Hard Sell* New York: Praeger

UNICEF (2007) *Child Poverty in Perspective: An Overview of Child Well-being in Rich Countries* Florence: UNICEF Innocenti Research Centre

Valentine, G. (2004) *Public Space and the Culture of Childhood* Aldershot: Ashgate

Vares, T. and Jackson, S. (2010) 'Preteen girls read "tween" popular culture: a contribution to the "sexualisation of girlhood" debates', paper presented at Child and Teen Consumption Conference, Linkoping, Sweden, June

Veblen, T. (1899/1975) *Theory of the Leisure Class* New York: Kelly

Vincent, C. and Ball, S. (2007) ' "Making up" the middle-class child: families, activities and class dispositions', *Sociology* 41(6): 1061–77

Wade, B. and Moore, M. (2000) *Baby Power: Give Your Child Real Learning Power* London: Egmont

Waerdahl, R. (2010) 'The dao of consumer socialisation: raising children in the Chinese consumer revolution', in D. Buckingham and V. Tingstad (eds.) *Childhood and Consumer Culture* London: Palgrave Macmillan

Wagg, S. (1992) 'One I made earlier: media, popular culture and the politics of childhood', in D. Strinati and S. Wagg *Come on Down! Popular Media Culture in Post-War Britain* London: Routledge

Walkerdine, V. (1997) *Daddy's Girl: Young Girls and Popular Culture* Basingstoke: Palgrave

Walkerdine, V. (1999) 'Violent boys and precocious girls: regulating childhood at the end of the millennium', *Contemporary Issues in Early Childhood* 1(1): 3–23

Waller, J. (1999) 'Free books for schools: an inquiry into the commercial sponsorship of school resource materials'. MA dissertation, University of Sheffield

Wang, Y. and Lobstein, T. (2006) 'Worldwide trends in childhood overweight and obesity', *International Journal of Pediatric Obesity* 1(1): 11–25

Ward, S. (1974) 'Consumer socialization', *Journal of Consumer Research* 1: 1–14

Warde, A. (1997) *Consumption, Food and Taste* London: Sage

Wasko, J. (2001) *Understanding Disney* Cambridge: Polity

Wasko, J. (2010) 'Online kids' sites: the latest commodification of children's culture', in D. Buckingham and V. Tingstad (eds.) *Childhood and Consumer Culture* London: Palgrave Macmillan

Weeks, J. (1981) *Sex, Politics and Society: The Regulation of Sexuality since 1800* London: Longman

Weeks, J. (2007) *The World We Have Won: The Remaking of Erotic and Intimate Life* London: Routledge

Wilkinson, G. (2006) 'Commercial breaks: an overview of corporate opportunities for commercialising education in US and English schools', *London Review of Education* 4(3): 253–69

Willett, R. (2004) 'The multiple identities of Pokémon fans', in J. Tobin (ed.) *Pikachu's Global Adventure: The Rise and Fall of Pokémon* Durham, NC: Duke University Press

Willett, R. (2008) 'Consumer citizens online: structure, agency and gender in online participation', in D. Buckingham (ed.) *Youth, Identity and Digital Media* Cambridge, MA: MIT Press. Open access edition www.mitpressjournals.org/toc/dmal/-/6

Williams, C. C. (2005) *A Commodified World? Mapping the Limits of Capitalism* London: Zed Books

Williams, C. L. (2006) *Inside Toyland: Working, Shopping and Social Inequality* Berkeley: University of California Press

Williams, R. (1976) *Keywords* Glasgow: Fontana

Willis, P. (1990) *Common Culture* Milton Keynes: Open University Press

Wolf, N. (1990) *The Beauty Myth* London: Chatto and Windus

Young, B. (1990) *Children and Television Advertising* Oxford: Oxford University Press

Young, B. (2003) *Advertising and Food Choice in Children* London: Food Advertising Unit, The Advertising Association

Young, B., Webley, P., Hetherington, M. and Zeedyk, S. (1996) *The Role of Television Advertising in Children's Food Choice* London: MAFF

Youth TGI (2008) BMRB report, cited in the Advertising Association report (2009) *Children's Wellbeing in a Commercial World* London: Advertising Association

Zelizer, V. (1985) *Pricing the Priceless Child: The Changing Social Value of Children* New York: Basic Books

Zelizer, V. (2002) 'Kids and commerce', *Childhood* 9(4): 375–96

Zhao, B. and Murdock, G. (1996) 'Little emperors: children and the making of Chinese consumerism', *Cultural Studies* 10(2): 201–17

Index